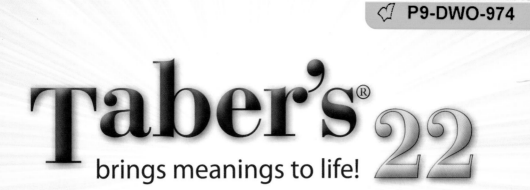
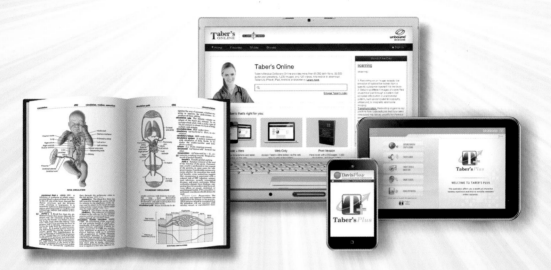
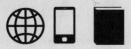
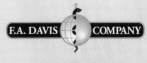

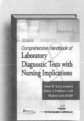
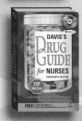
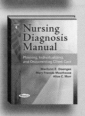
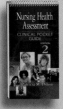

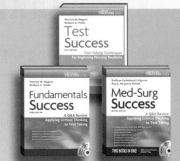
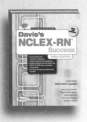
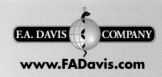

Case Studies in Nursing Fundamentals

■ MARGARET SORRELL TRUEMAN, RN, MSN, EdD, CNE

Fayetteville State University
Department of Nursing
Fayetteville, North Carolina

F.A. Davis Company • Philadelphia

F. A. DAVIS COMPANY
1915 Arch Street
Philadelphia, PA 19103
www.fadavis.com

Copyright © 2014 by F. A. Davis Company

Printed in the United States of America

Last digit indicates print number: 10 9 8 7 6 5 4 3 2 1

Publisher, Nursing: Lisa B. Houck
Director of Content Development: Darlene D. Pedersen
Project Editor: Jamie M. Elfrank
Electronic Project Editor: Katherine Crowley
Design and Illustration Manager: Carolyn O'Brien

As new scientific information becomes available through basic and clinical research, recommended treatments and drug therapies undergo changes. The author(s) and publisher have done everything possible to make this book accurate, up to date, and in accord with accepted standards at the time of publication. The author(s), editors, and publisher are not responsible for errors or omissions or for consequences from application of the book, and make no warranty, expressed or implied, in regard to the contents of the book. Any practice described in this book should be applied by the reader in accordance with professional standards of care used in regard to the unique circumstances that may apply in each situation. The reader is advised always to check product information (package inserts) for changes and new information regarding dose and contraindications before administering any drug. Caution is especially urged when using new or infrequently ordered drugs.

Library of Congress Cataloging-in-Publication Data

Trueman, Margaret Sorrell, author.
  Case studies in nursing fundamentals / Margaret Sorrell Trueman.
    p. ; cm.
  Includes bibliographical references and index.
  ISBN 978-0-8036-2923-3
  I. Title.
  [DNLM: 1. Nursing Care–Case Reports. 2. Nursing Process–Case Reports. WY 100.1]
  RT51
  610.73—dc23

                          2013043786

This book is dedicated to all the nursing students, past and present, who have touched my life. Their enthusiasm in learning all the new, exciting and sometimes frightening aspects of nursing has kept me on my toes, sustained my own passion for nursing, and made nursing education one of the most challenging and enjoyable times of my life. I thank you all.

Margaret (Peg) Sorrell Trueman earned a diploma in nursing from the Lankenau Hospital School of Nursing in Philadelphia, Pennsylvania, a bachelor of science degree in nursing from Queens University of Charlotte, Charlotte, North Carolina, a master's degree in nursing/adult health from the University of North Carolina at Charlotte and a Doctorate in Vocational and Technical Education from Clemson University, Clemson, South Carolina.

She has taught nursing in diploma, associate degree, baccalaureate, both pre-licensure and RN completion programs, and in master degree nursing programs. She has more than 30 years as a clinician in medical-surgical and critical care nursing and 25 years as a nurse educator. She has taught fundamentals of nursing, medical-surgical nursing, rehabilitation, critical care, pediatrics and the support courses of health assessment, pathophysiology, and research. She is a Certified Nurse Educator (CNE) through the National League of Nursing.

She is a member of the American Nurses Association, the North American Nursing Diagnosis Association-International and the American Heart Association. Her scholarship has been recognized in her membership in Sigma Theta Tau International and Epsilon Pi Tau, the international honor society for professions in technology. She has been recognized as one of the Great 100 Nurses of North Carolina. She has published in the areas of collaboration in practice and creative teaching techniques. Currently she is an Assistant Professor of Nursing at Fayetteville State University in Fayetteville, North Carolina.

I have been in nursing education over 25 years and the changes in the paradigms of teaching and testing have been both exhilarating and, at times, exasperating. Through all the changes, the nearly impossible question we have sought to answer has always been, "How do we truly teach the essence of real-life nursing decision-making in a safe way without spending millions of dollars?"

I'd like to say I brilliantly discovered one possible solution to this question, but I have to confess that the impetus for making fundamentals of nursing come alive came from my daughter, a kindergarten teacher, who in a moment of Zen, watching me put together lecture after lecture after lecture commented . . . Isn't it a shame that adult learners do not get to play and learn like my kindergarteners . . and my AH-HA! moment struck and I thought: note to self —let the students play with the information we want them to learn and the beginning of the idea for the use of the case method in the Fundamentals of Nursing began . . .

The goal of this book is not in the presentation of information for nursing care; many books already exist for this purpose but rather to facilitate an understanding and ability to use the information in real-life nursing practice situations. This book is to help students not only learn the information vital to nursing practice but also to facilitate an ability to use the learned information in real-life clinical settings encountered in everyday nursing practice. Nursing is a participation sport and requires not only the understanding of the rules and regulations of the sport but the ability to play the skills within a framework of teamwork and optimal outcomes, for both the clients for whom we care and for the nursing profession itself.

Case learning is not a new concept; teaching through storytelling has been around since the beginning of time. What is more modern is its use in a structured manner to enhance learning outcomes when the goal is that of safe and successful application of learned information. The method of case-based instruction is credited to Christopher Columbus Langdell, a law professor and later Dean of the Harvard Law School in the late 1800s. He believed that the most realistic way to study law was to examine and work through real-life legal situations. He used appellate court cases and decisions to prepare students for the real world of legal practice (William, 1992).

For nursing education, learning based on situations commonly encountered in clinical practice helps students develop the knowledge and know-how for implementation of safe nursing care. Cases present a high-frequency, low-stake learning modality that can mimic real care situations. They allow exposure to different care situations that often, as a result of limited clinical resources commonly encountered in programs of nursing, are not available as real-time experiences for nursing students.

In general, cases encourage students to think about practice and support the development of critical thinking skills. By changing the focus from content to process, the active learning of nursing practice becomes the charge to student learners rather than the responsibility of the faculty. Ownership of outcomes, a thrust of nursing practice in the interactional process in client care, becomes the foundation of not only the learning of nursing practice but a foundation tool of the practice

Research indicates that students feel that case studies add significant realism to their learning because of the relevancy to the course concepts and they are more engaged when cases are integrated into the instruction (Hofsten, Gustafsson, &Haggstrom, 2010; Yadav, Shaver & Meckl, 2010). The charge to faculty, in the presentation of concepts, and the charge to students, in their learning of concepts, is that the knowledge must be used, not just acquired. To this end, case-based instruction provides the ability to make teaching/learning an active process instead of a passive one.

Organized by the major concepts addressed in foundational courses in nursing, the case studies support the remembering, understanding, application, and analysis of the information. As educators recognize and students come to learn, case method integrates Blooms taxonomy, the format entrenched in the teaching and testing of nursing practice. Frequently educators see nursing students bring to their nursing studies a rich skill base in the memorization and recall of knowledge. However, making the quantum leap across the divide to the application of that knowledge has led to some not-so-successful outcomes in students who were felt to have the prerequisite skills needed for success in nursing education. Case-method instruction supports the use of the information presented in each concept across the domains of learning as well as structured within the nursing process. Facilitating the student's ability to manipulate their knowledge and growing practice base across all uses of information helps them integrate the foundational concepts of nursing practice inherent to every nursing situation.

The purpose of case studies as presented in this textbook is to:

1. Present the foundational knowledge needed in situational decision making
2. Provide true-to-life patient-care situations that require application and analysis of learned information to ensure safe and competent decision making in patient care
3. Make the learning of nursing REAL

Terry Delpier (2006) in explaining the applicability of case studies in nursing education so eloquently states, cases are the best way to teach nursing students how to think like nurses (p. 209).

For students, this textbook provides the opportunity to play with the knowledge gained in regard to nursing practice at the fundamental level. The author also recognizes that though the learning of the safe application of nursing practice is the pinnacle of your education, that success on the NCLEX-RN® licensure examination is of equal importance. The ability to develop, maintain, and safely apply the concepts of nursing practice is quantified by your ability to be successful on comprehensive examinations throughout your course of study; and in essence be successful on the mother of all comprehensive examinations, the licensure examination. Case-based learning is an important strategy towards this end. Students exposed to case-based learning methods were found to score significantly better on comprehensive examinations than those students not afforded the opportunity of this learning method (Beers & Bowden, 2005; Pariseau & Kezim, 2007).

I hope you enjoy the reading and use of the book as I certainly enjoyed writing the stories. The stories are a reflection and composite of the many clients I have had the pleasure of meeting and the privilege of being a part of their stories in their journeys through the healthcare system; a system which nursing is the pivotal aspect of their successful outcomes.

PEG SORRELL TRUEMAN

Beers, G. W., & Bowden, S. (2005). The effect of teaching method on long-term knowledge retention. *Journal of Nursing Education, 44,* 511–514.

Delpier, T. (2006). CASES 101: Learning to teach with cases. *Nursing Education Perspectives,27,* 204–209.

Herreid, C. F. (1997). What makes a good case? Some basic rules of good storytelling help teachers generate excitement in class. *Journal of College Science Teaching, 27,* 163–165.

Hofsten, A., Gustafsson, C., & Haggstrom, E. (2010). Case seminars open doors to deeper understanding—nursing students' experiences of learning. *Nurse Education Today, 30,* 533–538.

Paruseau, S., & Kezim, B. (2007). The effect of using case studies in business statistics. *Journal of Education for Business, 83* (1), 27–31.

William, S. M. (1992). Putting case-based instruction into context: Examples from legal and medical education.*The Journal of Learning Sciences, 2,* 367–427.

Yadav, A., Shaver, G. N., & Meckl, P. (2010). Lessons learned: Implementing case teaching method in a mechanical engineering course. *Journal of Engineering Education, 99*(1), 55–63.

SHERYL ALLEN, PHDC, MSN, RN
ADN Faculty
Meridian Community College
Meridian, Mississippi

RITA C. BERGEVIN, RN-BC, MA, CWCN
Clinical Associate Professor
Binghamton University, Decker School of Nursing
Binghamton, New York

DONNA BEUK, MSN, RN, CNE
Assistant Professor
Auburn University at Montgomery
Montgomery, Alabama

STACI M. BORUFF, PhD(c), MSN, RN
Associate Professor of Nursing
Walters State Community College
Morristown, Tennessee

LAURIE S. DE GROOT, BSN, MSN, RN, GCNS-BC
Program Leader and Nursing Instructor
Associate Degree Nursing Program
North Iowa Area Community College
Mason City, Iowa

DEBORAH DYE, RN, MSN
Nursing Department Chair
Ivy Tech Community College
Lafayette, Indiana

JAMIE FIELDS, MS, RN
Instructor of Nursing
Eastern Oklahoma State College
Idabel, Oklahoma

MARGARET FRIED, RN, MA
Instructional Faculty
Pima Community College
Tucson, Arizona

YOLANDA B. HALL, RN, MSN
Professor, Vocational Nursing
Austin Community College
Austin, Texas

SUSAN J. HAYDEN, RN, PhD
Assistant Professor
University of South Alabama
Mobile, Alabama

PAM HAYS, RN, MSN
Associate Professor, Nursing
John A. Logan College
Carterville, Illinois

JUDY R. HEMBD, RN, MSN
Professor of Nursing
Collin College
McKinney, Texas

TERESA V. HURLEY, DHED, MS, RN
Associate Professor of Nursing
Mount Saint Mary College
Newburgh, New York

SHIRLEY JEANDRON, RN, MSN, MBA
Nursing Instructor
Delgado-Charity School of Nursing
New Orleans, Louisana

PATRICIA T. KETCHAM, RN, MSN
Director of Nursing Laboratories
Oakland University, School of Nursing
Rochester, Minnesota

ROSEMARY MACY, PhD, RN
Associate Professor
Boise State University
Boise, Idaho

KASSIE MCKENNY, MSN, RN, CNE
Assistant Professor
Clarkson College
Omaha, Nebraska

JOSEPH MOLINATTI, EdD, RN
Assistant Professor of Nursing
College of Mount Saint Vincent
Bronx, New York

SUSAN L. PATTERSON, RN, MS, CCM, CNE
Faculty, School of Nursing
Carolinas College of Health Sciences
Charlotte, North Carolina

JANICE PODWIKA, RN, BSN, MS
Faculty
Maricopa Community College
Phoenix, Arizona

PHYLLIS ROWE, DNP, RN, ANP
Professor Emerita, Nursing
Riverside City College
Riverside, California

DIANE J. SHEETS, MS, RN, CNS
Clinical Instructor
Ohio State University College of Nursing
Columbus, Ohio

AMANDA SIMMONS, MSN, RN
Nursing Faculty
Technical College of the Lowcountry
Beaufort, South Carolina

JUDY STAUDER, MSN, RN
Assistant Professor
Stark State College
North Canton, Ohio

LINDA D. WAGNER, EdD, MSN, RN
Professor and Chairperson, Department of Nursing
Central Connecticut State University
New Britain, Connecticut

AMY WEAVER, MSN, RN, ACNS-BC
Instructor
Youngtown State University
Youngstown, Ohio

KHATAZA JESSIE WHEATLEY, RN, MSN
Assistant Professor-BSN Program
University of Arkansas at Fort Smith
Fort Smith, Arkansas

RYAN YOUNG, RN, MSN
Assistant Professor of Nursing
State University of New York (SUNY) Canton
Canton, New York

No great endeavor is ever accomplished in a silo. So many people contributed to the development and completion of this textbook. First I would like to thank my team at F.A. Davis for their encouragement and support through the entire production process:

Greg Spradley (Representative) for giving me the opportunity to pursue my dream of authorship.

Lisa Houck (Publisher) for your support and feedback as I navigated all the challenges of writing and producing a textbook.

Jamie Elfrank (Project Editor) for your advice and direction throughout the details of putting together this project.

Lastly, and pivotal to my team, was the mentorship and coaching I received from Judith Wilkinson. At the beginning of this project, it was her textbook that gave rise to the idea of a conceptually driven case-method textbook for Fundamentals. Being able to speak with her, (understanding that this was a neophyte speaking with a Guru— I was so nervous!) I gained advice and direction, and most importantly, had someone who had complete faith in my ability to bring-to-life the intricacies of nursing practice.

I thank my family for their support as so much time was spent thinking and doing to bring this book to fruition.

To my friends, who never wavered in their awe that someone they knew was writing a book, I am grateful for the confidence you had in me and I can finally say, yes—the book is finally a reality.

To Michele who has been a gift in my life and whose support kept me grounded and working through the tough times; it was her never-ending patience, listening to me vent, and her great words of wisdom; and to Team 4, the heart and fist I needed for those days when I doubted my ability to write at all.

Last to Baby B: Patty—I could never do all that I have done in my life without your unwavering love, support, and belief in me.

Contents

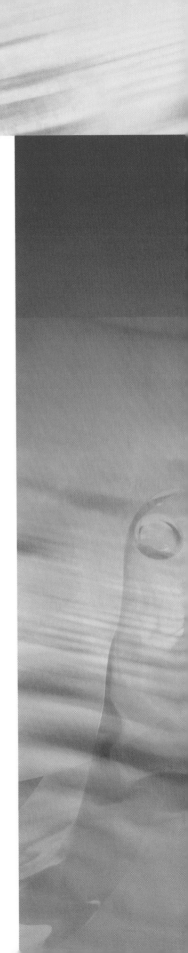

UNIT 1 The Theory and Application
of Nursing Practice

The Nursing Profession and Practice	1
Critical Thinking and the Nursing Process	19
Nursing Process *Assessment*	31
Nursing Process *Nursing Diagnosis*	43
Nursing Process *Planning Outcomes*	57
Nursing Process *Planning Interventions*	65
Nursing Process *Evaluation*	73
Nursing Process *Implementation*	79
Nursing Theory	87
Research	91

UNIT 2 Factors Affecting Health

Growth and Development	95
Health and Illness	105
Psychosocial Health and Illness	111
Family	119
Culture and Ethnicity	127
Spirituality	135
Loss, Grief and Dying	141

UNIT 3 Essential Nursing Interventions

Documenting and Reporting	149
Vital Signs	157
Communication and Therapeutic Relationships	165
Health Assessment	171
Promoting Asepsis and Preventing Infection	177
Safety *Falls*	187

Self-Care Ability *Hygiene*   193
Medication Administration   201
Teaching and Learning   211

UNIT 4 Supporting Physiological Functioning

Stress-Coping-Adaptation   219
Nutrition   227
Elimination *Urinary*   235
Bowel Elimination *Constipation*   243
Bowel Elimination *Diarrhea*   247
Sensory Perception   249
Pain Management   253
Activity and Exercise   261
Sexual Health   269
Sleep and Rest   275
Skin Integrity   279
Oxygenation   287
Perfusion   293
Fluid, Electrolyte, and Acid-Base Balance   297

UNIT 5 Nursing Functions

Leading and Management   305
Informatics   317
Holism   323
Health Promotion   327

UNIT 6 Context for Nurses' Work

Perioperative Nursing   331
Community-Based Care   341
Ethics and Values   349
Legal Issues   357

Index   363

Theory and Application of Nursing Practice

The Nursing Profession and Practice

Before reading the chapter, write a short two-paragraph narrative defining and describing your personal perspective on the question "What is nursing and what do nurses do?" Set it aside while you work through the content that presents the evolution and practice of nursing as an integral part of the healthcare delivery system.

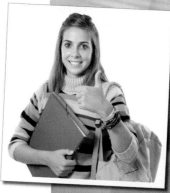

Mary Jane had been accepted into a nursing program and excitedly announced it to a group of people at church. She received a mixture of comments regarding her desire to become a nurse including the following:

- "You must really have a special calling to help the sick."
- "Gonna catch you a rich doctor-husband?"
- "Going to join the war on illness and diseases, are you?"
- "You will get to help the doctors do all their hard work."
- "Oh my—I could not give shots all day; you have to be a little mean."

1. Discuss the perception of nursing portrayed by each comment within the historical context associated with the profession of nursing.

Content	Historical Context
"You must really have a special calling to help the sick."	
"Gonna catch you a rich doctor-husband?"	
"Going to join the war on illness and diseases, are you?"	

Content	Historical Context
"You will get to help the doctors do all their hard work."	
"Oh my—I could not give shots all day; you have to be a little mean."	

2. Describe the two images commonly associated with Florence Nightingale, the founder of modern nursing.

_____

_____

_____

_____

_____

_____

3. Florence Nightingale exhibited the characteristics of a "full-spectrum nurse." Discuss each component inherent to the thinking roles of the nurse and how they were integral to Florence Nightingale's major contribution to the profession of standards to control the spread of disease in hospitals.

_____

_____

_____

_____

_____

_____

_____

_____

_____

_____

_____

_____

_____

_____

_____

_____

_____

Thinking Roles	Standards to Control the Spread of Disease in Hospitals

4. Gender, race, and ethnicity are changing the "face" of nursing. Looking at your own cohort of nursing students, does the composition of your group reflect the *2012 National Sample Survey of Registered Nurses*? Within your own community of learners, how can your program increase the diversity of the nursing profession?

_____

_____

_____

_____

_____

_____

_____

_____

_____

_____

_____

_____

_____

_____

_____

_____

_____

_____

_____

_____

_____

_____

_____

_____

_____

_____

_____

_____

_____

Nursing has been defined by many entities throughout history but it is of vital importance to clearly articulate what nursing is and what nurses do within the context of the ever-changing nature of nursing, healthcare, and society.

5. Why is it so important for the nursing profession to have a clear definition?

_____

_____

_____

_____

_____

_____

_____

_____

_____

_____

_____

6. The International Council of Nurses (ICN), the American Nurses Association (ANA), and the Canadian Nurses Association (CNA) have delineated definitions for the profession. What are the similarities and differences among these definitions of nursing?

_____

_____

_____

_____

_____

_____

_____

_____

_____

_____

_____

_____

_____

_____

_____

_____

_____

Key Term/Concept	ICN	ANA	CNA

Key Term/Concept	ICN	ANA	CNA

7. What are the ANA essential features of professional nursing? Should they be included as key concepts in the ANA's definition of professional nursing?

_____

_____

_____

_____

_____

_____

_____

_____

_____

_____

_____

_____

_____

_____

_____

_____

_____

_____

_____

8. Describe the roles and functions of the nurse. Give an example of how you, as a nursing student, can operationalize these roles in some manner. *Note*: not all roles may be within the scope of your nursing student practice.

Roles and Functions of the Nurse	
Role and Function	**Examples**

Roles and Functions of the Nurse—cont'd

Role and Function	Examples

9. Outline the three descriptors of this career called nursing: a profession, a discipline, and an occupation.

_____

_____

_____

_____

_____

_____

_____

_____

_____

_____

_____

_____

_____

_____

_____

_____

_____

_____

_____

_____

_____

_____

_____

_____

_____

_____

_____

Now let's return to your brief narrative describing your own perspective on the question "What is nursing and what do nurses do?" and address the following:

10. Which historical influences are reflected in your description?

_____

11. Which professional organization's definition best reflects your own description of nursing? Explain.

_____

_____

_____

12. Identify the roles reflected in your own description of nursing.

_____

13. Discuss which descriptor of nursing is best reflected in your own description of nursing.

_____

_____

_____

_____

_____

_____

Nurses' educational options to meet the initial requirements for licensure are a much-debated topic within the profession.

14. Discuss the five educational pathways leading to licensure as a registered nurse (RN).

_____

_____

_____

_____

_____

_____

_____

_____

_____

_____

_____

_____

_____

_____

_____

_____

15. Were you aware of the other pathways available for the study of nursing? Why did you choose your present program of study for RN licensure?

_____

_____

_____

_____

16. What is "continuing education" and why is it vital to your nursing practice?

_____

_____

_____

_____

_____

As a part of the educational sphere of nursing, socialization is the informal education that occurs as you move into the new profession.

17. Describe the ways that socialization occurs within this informal process. How does this process integrate into your current course of study? Give examples.

_____

_____

_____

_____

---

18. Describe each of the stages of Benner's model pertaining to the acquisition of clinical skills and judgment.

Skill Level	Description of Skill

19. It is recognized that a new graduate usually functions at the Stage 2: Advanced Beginner level. Is it appropriate to expect this level of functioning as an exit competency for your program of study? Explain.

Nursing practice is regulated by laws and guided by standards of practice.

20. What are the differences between the intent of the laws regulating nursing practice and the standards guiding nursing practice?

_____

_____

_____

_____

_____

_____

_____

_____

_____

_____

_____

21. How do practicing nurses, professional nursing organizations, and other professions use the standards of practice? How can you use them within your own scope of practice as a nursing student?

_____

_____

_____

_____

_____

_____

_____

_____

_____

_____

Nursing is supported by many nursing organizations that work to establish standards of practice, ensure educational standards, and ensure quality of nursing care in all practice settings.

22. Discuss how the ANA/CNA, the National League for Nursing (NLN), and the ICN are all needed to ensure global standards for the profession of nursing.

_____

_____

_____

_____

_____

_____

_____

_____

_____

_____

_____

_____

_____

_____

Nursing encompasses a spectrum of care and addresses the continuum of human health needs from health promotion to end-of-life care in a variety of practice settings. Within this spectrum of care there are many trends, both societal and those within nursing and healthcare, that are affecting contemporary nursing practice.

23. Discuss the four purposes of nursing care within the continuum of human health needs.

Purpose	Range of Services

24. For each of the following practice settings, give examples of activities that may occur within the continuum of human health needs. You may need to refer to other chapters in your textbook that address particular practice settings.
   a. Extended care facilities
   b. Ambulatory care
   c. Home care
   d. Community health

Continuum of Human Health Needs	Extended Care	Ambulatory Care	Home Care	Community Health
Health Promotion				
Illness Prevention				
Health Restoration				
End-of-Life Care				

25. Discuss each of the following societal and healthcare trends and the possible impact, both positive and negative, on the purposes of nursing care:
   a. National economy
   b. Aging population
   c. Roles of the healthcare consumer
   d. Complementary and alternative medicine
   e. Use of nursing assistive personnel (NAP)

_____

_____

_____

_____

_____

_____

_____

_____

_____

_____

_____

_____

_____

_____

Critical Thinking and the Nursing Process

The components of nursing practice include doing, caring, and thinking. Much of what is recognized about nursing reflects the "doing" component, the activities that make up the practice, along with the caring component. The third component, thinking, is the foundational concept that is essential to all aspects of nursing care.

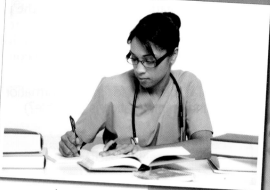

Heaslip (1992) defines critical thinking as the method for clinical decision making; it is "the ability to think in a systematic and logical manner with openness to questions and to reflect on the reasoning process used to ensure safe nursing practice and quality care."

1. Identify and give a personal definition of the key concepts in Heaslip's definition of critical thinking.

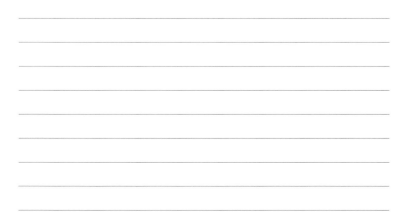

18. What is the nursing process and how does it support nursing's practical knowledge?

_____

_____

_____

19. List the phases of the nursing process and give a three- or four-word descriptor of each phase.

_____

_____

_____

_____

_____

_____

_____

_____

_____

_____

_____

_____

20. Explain how critical thinking and the nursing process are interrelated.

_____

_____

21. Why is caring a vital part of the nursing profession's theoretical and practical knowledge?

_____

_____

_____

_____

22. In the following patient care situation, describe nursing actions that demonstrate the five components of caring:

■ Renee is a 21-year-old female patient on the rehabilitation unit who is recovering from injuries that resulted in paralysis from her waist down. She is a junior honor student at the university, a member of the soccer team, and an active member of her church choir. She is struggling with learning how to deal with her loss of mobility.

The four major concepts that describe full-spectrum nursing—thinking, doing, caring, and patient situation—provide a model for professional practice.

23. Describe the main concepts inherent in the nurse-patient dyad and how they work together to facilitate positive patient outcomes.

Reference

Heaslip, P. (1992). *Creating the thinking practitioner: Critical thinking in clinical practice*. Kamloops, BC: University College of the Cariboo. (ERIC Document Reproduction Service No. ED 354-822)

Nursing Process: Assessment

Assessment is the first step of the nursing process and it provides the data that allow the nurse to help the patient. It is a systematic gathering of information related to the physical, mental, spiritual, socioeconomic, and cultural status of the individual. Let's look at a patient situation common in the healthcare system.

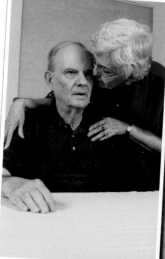

■ Mr. Robert McClelland, an 81-year-old, is a new admission from the local hospital to your long-term care facility. After Mr. McClelland's last bout with pneumonia and congestive heart failure, his wife of 59 years has decided she is no longer able to care for him at home. Mrs. McClelland states, "He has just gotten too weak and can't help me care for him. I am so afraid he will fall and hurt himself. I am so worn out trying to care for him myself. I have to bathe him and remind him to eat; sometimes I've had to feed him myself or he won't eat. He can be so forgetful. I hope I am making the right decision for him, because he never wanted to go into a nursing home."

1. Why is your admission assessment foundational to the care of Mr. McClelland?

_____

_____

_____

2. Describe the four features of assessment and why they are critical to ensuring positive outcomes within the context of interdisciplinary care for Mr. McClelland.

_____

_____

_____

_____

_____

_____

_____

_____

_____

_____

3. Describe how assessment is essential to the other steps of the nursing process.

_____

_____

_____

_____

_____

_____

_____

_____

_____

_____

_____

_____

4. Using The American Nurses Association *Standards of Practice*, identify the key concepts/phrases within Standard 1 characteristic to a comprehensive database. Categorize these concepts within the model of full-spectrum nursing.

Key Concept/Phrase	Concept of the Model

You are preparing to complete an initial comprehensive assessment with Mr. McClelland. This will include both the nursing history interview and the observation/physical examination.

5. Identify all primary and secondary sources of information that you could use to help gather information about this patient. Differentiate the types of data that can be elicited from these sources.

_____

_____

_____

_____

6. Which special needs assessments, a type of focused assessment, are indicated at this time? Discuss the data that support your decision.

_____

_____

_____

_____

15. Discuss the implications of failing to validate your conclusion regarding these data on the nursing plan of care.

_____

_____

_____

_____

_____

Once completed, a comprehensive assessment provides a wealth of information about the patient. It is then important to bring together these data within an organizing framework to facilitate prioritization and completeness of the data. Organizing data helps you cluster data and find patterns that will guide you in clinical decision making.

16. Categorize the following data elicited from Mr. and Mrs. McClelland during the comprehensive assessment using Maslow's Hierarchy of Needs (non-nursing model) and Gordon's Functional Health Patterns (nursing model).

Datum	Maslow	Gordon*

17. Looking at the clusters of data for each model, identify one advantage of each model in developing a plan of care for this patient.

_____

_____

_____

_____

18. Using the clusters of data, recognize the abnormal data within the patterns and then identify two top problem areas for Mr. McClelland. How did you come to this conclusion?

_____

_____

_____

_____

_____

_____

_____

_____

_____

_____

_____

_____

The documentation of assessment data, both initial and ongoing, benefits patients and the healthcare team by providing access to information for effective patient care.

19. How does the documentation of data provide continuity throughout the nursing process?

_____

_____

_____

_____

_____

_____

_____

You are reviewing the following documentation regarding the discharge and transfer of Mr. McClelland to your long-term care facility for information relevant to the development of the plan of care.

■ 81 y.o. male appears ready for d/c and transfer to LTCF accompanied by his wife. No respiratory distress noted at this time and patient said his breathing seems ok. No oxygen therapy needed for transport. Integumentary WNL. Pt. seems agreeable to placement. Wife is anxious about his well-being in regard to eating and ambulating safely. Apetite has been good. Does need assistance to go to the barhroom. IVL d/c'd.

20. Using the guidelines for recording assessment data, identify the inaccuracies in this document and rewrite it to reflect professional documentation. You may add information as needed to meet a guideline but the final note must reflect the status of the patient at time of admission to your long-term care facility. You may use the data provided in the scenario and in question 16.

As follow-up to any assessment it is important to reflect critically about the assessment. As you gain confidence and competency in assessment, questions used to guide your assessment will become a natural response to your assessment process.

21. Why is it important to the nurse, to the patient, and to the healthcare team that you reflect critically about your patient assessments?

Nursing Process: Nursing Diagnosis

During this phase of the nursing process you will analyze the assessment data obtained on Mr. McClelland upon admission to your long-term care facility to identify his health status, including strengths, problems, and factors contributing to the problems. An abbreviated admission database is provided for you to facilitate your work through the diagnostic process and formation of the pertinent nursing diagnoses for Mr. McClelland.

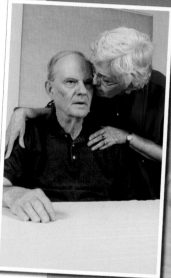

1. Why is the diagnostic phase of the nursing process critical to the development of the plan of care?

_____

_____

_____

_____

2. Explain how nursing diagnoses and the use of nursing diagnostic labels help validate nursing as a profession.

_____

_____

_____

_____

_____

_____

_____

_____

_____

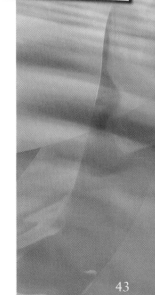

In the identification of health problems, the decision about how the problem will be addressed drives the type of diagnosis (nursing, medical, or collaborative) that the problem receives.

3. From the database obtained at admission, Mr. McClelland has an identified health problem of "forgetfulness." His medical diagnosis is early-onset dementia. Based on the definitions, discuss how the nursing diagnoses can be determined from the health issue of "forgetfulness" and the collaborative problems from the medical diagnosis of dementia.

4. How could the use of the medical diagnosis to determine appropriate nursing diagnoses be detrimental to Mr. McClelland's plan of care?

5. Describe the five types of nursing diagnoses that may be identified for a patient.

_____

_____

_____

_____

_____

_____

_____

_____

_____

_____

_____

_____

_____

_____

_____

6. Utilizing Mr. McClelland's admission assessment, identify assessment findings that may represent each type of status of nursing diagnosis. You may need to use available references to determine the significance of data listed on the admission database.

Type	Example of Data from Admission Assessment	
	Subjective Data	Objective Data
Actual		
Potential		
Possible*		

(Continued)

Type	Example of Data from Admission Assessment	
Syndrome*		
Wellness (Health Promotion)		

Through diagnostic reasoning, you will critically think through the data to determine the holistic needs of the patient so that a plan of care can be developed and implemented.

7. Referring to the listing of "Recognizing Cues," analyze the data provided on the admission assessment. Highlight/underline the significant data (cues) about Mr. McClelland. Label each finding with the appropriate cue.

_____

_____

_____

_____

_____

_____

_____

_____

_____

_____

_____

Recognizing Cues

The following may indicate cues.

A deviation from population norms

Example: For a well-conditioned athlete who is not a smoker, a heart rate of 120 beats per minute would probably be an unhealthy response (cue). But remember that in addition, you must always consider whether the response is normal for the patient or the situation.

Recognizing Cues—cont'd

Changes in usual health patterns are not explained by developmental or situational changes

Example: What change has Todd (Meet Your Patient) experienced in the 3 days before admission to the ED? Is there any developmental or situational explanation for his decreased sensation and mobility? No. It is an unhealthy response: a cue.

Indications of delayed growth and development

Example: A 17-year-old girl has not yet experienced menses, her breasts are just barely developed, and she has very scant pubic and underarm hair.

Changes in usual behaviors in roles or relationships

Example: During her first year at college, a previously successful student begins to skip classes. She stays up late partying and sleeps most of the day. She no longer keeps in contact with her friends, and despite a previous close relationship with her parents, she barely talks to them when they telephone.

Nonproductive or dysfunctional behavior

This may or may not be a change in behavior. It could be a long-standing dysfunctional behavior. *Example:* A man has been abusing alcohol for many years, even though it is causing many problems with his family and job and has begun to damage his liver.

Source: Adapted from Gordon, M. (1994). *Nursing diagnosis: Process and application* (3rd ed.). St. Louis, MO: C. V. Mosby.

8. Where do the identified data "cluster" in Mr. McClelland's database?

_____

_____

_____

_____

_____

_____

_____

_____

_____

_____

_____

_____

_____

_____

_____

_____

9. Identify data gaps or inconsistencies. Data gaps are often the information needed to clarify the presence of a health problem. Often gaps are related to the defining characteristics (what further information would validate the problem) or the etiology (the cause of the problem). Develop two questions you would ask Mr. and Mrs. McClelland to resolve these gaps or inconsistencies.

Data Gap	Inconsistency

10. For each cluster of data, make a conclusion about the patient's health status using one of the following labels: strength, wellness, actual problem, or potential problem.

11. For each labeled data cluster, identify an appropriate nursing diagnostic label.

_____

_____

_____

_____

_____

_____

_____

_____

_____

_____

_____

_____

_____

12. Identify the possible etiological factors for each diagnostic label that you identified from the data. (See next table.)

Diagnostic Label*	Etiological Factors

Diagnostic Label	Etiological Factors

13. Why is this identification of etiological factors so important in the development of the plan of care?

_____

_____

_____

14. Discuss the importance of verifying the identified problems and contributing factors with the patient.

_____

_____

_____

_____

_____

_____

_____

_____

15. Prioritize your list of problems by needs theory and problem urgency. Discuss your rationale for the manner in which you prioritized the list.

_____

_____

_____

_____

Rationale: Maslow's Needs Theory	Diagnostic Label	Problem Urgency
Physiological		
Safety & Security		
Love & Belonging		
Self-Esteem		
Cognitive		
Self-Actualization		

16. How can patient preference impact the ranking of the identified problems?

_____

_____

_____

_____

_____

Reflection of your diagnostic reasoning is vital to ensuring accurate nursing diagnoses for each patient. As a student you have developed a sound background in the biological and psychosocial sciences as well as an understanding of the cultural and spiritual domains of humanness.

17. Discuss how your own self-knowledge can negatively impact your diagnostic reasoning.

_____

_____

_____

_____

_____

_____

_____

_____

18. Using the NANDA-I Taxonomy II: Domains, Classes and Diagnoses (Labels), write a three-part statement for the three actual diagnoses of highest priority, a two-part statement for the two at-risk diagnoses, and a statement for the wellness diagnosis for Mr. McClelland.

Keys to the parts of a diagnostic statement:

- The nursing diagnostic label is a description of the human response to a health problem and drives the goals of the plan of care.
- Etiologies are the factors that cause, contribute to, or create a risk for the problem and may include a NANDA-I label, defining characteristics, related to or risk factors. The etiology individualizes the plan of care because it directed the nursing interventions; choose the etiologies that are "fixable" or influenced by nursing interventions.
- Defining characteristics describe the information that describes the presence of the human response and are data (subjective and objective) directly assessed from the patient.

_____

_____

_____

_____

_____

_____

_____

_____

_____

_____

_____

_____

_____

19. Identify one collaborative problem indicated by Mr. McClelland's medical diagnosis.

_____

_____

20. Using the guidelines for judging the quality of diagnostic statements, critique the five nursing diagnostic statements you wrote to reflect the priority issues for the plan of care for Mr. McClelland. List the corrections that were indicated in regard to:
a. Appropriateness of the NANDA-I label

_____

_____

_____

b. Clear cause and effect between the etiology and the problem

_____

_____

c. The etiologies contributing to the problem do not simply restate the NANDA-I label.

_____

d. Use of medical diagnoses or treatments as etiological factors

_____

_____

_____

e. Clear, professional language

_____

f. Concise statement

_____

g. Descriptive and specific

_____

_____

h. Nursing diagnostic label is a patient (human) response
i. Use of judgmental language

_____

j. Legally questionable language

_____

_____

_____

_____

21. One of the criticisms of the NANDA-I system proposes that there should not be any standardized language to describe nursing knowledge and nursing work. Discuss from a nursing student perspective why standardization supports your learning of the profession.

_____

_____

_____

_____

_____

_____

Admission Data Base: Resident: Mr. McClelland

SUBJECTIVE SOURCE(S): _RESIDENT AND SPOUSE_	OBJECTIVE
Health Perception–Health Management Pattern Reason for seeking health care: _Wife can no longer care for resident at home._ Health rating: _Fair_ Perception of illness: Resident states: _I am doing just fine—I am being treated like I can't take care of things._ Spouse states: _It has really affected him—he has to be bathed and reminded to eat._	**Overall Physical Appearance** _Aware of surroundings, needs reminding of now being at the facility and not still at the hospital. Sitting upright in chair at bedside, facial expressions appropriate to verbal context._ **Allergies** _Latex (difficulty breathing)_ _Penicillin (hives, itching)_
Nutritional–Metabolic Pattern Daily food and fluid intake Breakfast: _Best meal of the day 90%–100%_ _Usually eggs, toast, juice, coffee. I like bacon but they won't let me have it._ Lunch: _50% usually sandwiches and iced tea. I like potato chips but they won't let me have them_ Supper: _I am not a supper eater. I get enough to eat—she always puts too much food on my plate_ Snack: _He snacks on cookies a lot—he has a sweet tooth._ Effect of illnesses on food intake: _I get out of breath half way through my meal_ _Without salt, food doesn't taste good so why bother eating?_ Skin condition: _It's always dry and flakey._ Nail condition: _Spouse states, "He needs a podiatrist to look at his toes."_ Difficulty gaining/losing weight: Spouse: _He has lost weight. I have to remind him to eat. He doesn't eat enough—he always leaves food on his plate. I don't think he's getting enough to eat._	**Height** 76 inches **Weight** 137# **BMI:** 16.7 **Temp:** 97.8°F (oral) **Skin:** _Pale, cool to touch, dry with tenting present, brownish discoloration noted to both lower extremities from the knee down to the foot._ **Nails:** _Pale in color, spoon-shaped with clubbing, thickened toenails._ **Oral Mucosa:** _Pale, intact, no lesions, upper and lower dentures present._
Elimination Pattern Bowel habits: _I had a bowel movement this morning, I usually go every day. It is normal for me, it's brown and formed. If I have trouble I take some milk of magnesia._ Bladder habits: _I usually need to go 6–7x/day, I go a lot because I take a water pill which also makes it real light in color. I usually have to get up once or twice a night and if I can't get to the bathroom fast enough I have an accident. It seems that is happening more and more lately._	**Abdomen:** _Flat, soft with active bowel sounds in all four quadrants._ **Bladder:** _Voiding small amounts light yellow urine with some sediment noted._
Activity–Exercise Pattern Daily activities Hygiene: _Spouse: "He gets washed up every morning and I give him a total bath once a week."_ Leisure activities: _I like to watch TV and I used to like reading the morning paper but it seems like it's just gotten too long to read._ Occupation: _Retired from local utility company, management level._ Effect of illness on activity: _I am just fine getting up and doing for myself. I don't like it but she will insist that she help me with my bath._	**Respiratory:** _Respirations 24/minute regular and unlabored. Oxygen saturation 92% on room air. Lungs sounds with bibasilar crackles, no cough present._ **Cardiovascular:** _Apical pulse 87 bpm and regular. BP pressure in right arm 160/86, left arm 158/84. Peripheral pulses palpable with pedal and post tibial pulses weak bilaterally. 2+ pitting edema notes in feet and ankles bilaterally._ **Musculoskeletal:** _Gait unsteady, posture slightly stooped when standing, no compromise noted in ROM though weakness to all extremities._

Admission Data Base: Resident: Mr. McClelland (cont'd)

SUBJECTIVE	OBJECTIVE
Sleep–Rest Pattern <u>Sleep characteristics</u>: *I get about 5–6 hrs/night depending on how often I have to pee. Once that happens I have difficulty getting back to sleep and remaining asleep—seems my bladder never sleeps. Also I wear oxygen at night and sometimes that bothers me enough to keep me from resting well.*	**Appearance:** *Yawning intermittently, impatient with interview questions.*
Sensory–Perceptual Pattern <u>Perceptions of senses</u>: *I see ok as long as I have my glasses and I have these hearing aids in my ears which helps me hear everything. I can taste and smell ok and I don't really have any pain to speak of.*	**Visual Exam:** *Presence of glasses, EOMs intact, PERRLA at 3mm bilaterally.* **Hearing:** *External canal clean with no lesions, difficulty understanding all words spoken to him in the interview.*
Cognitive Pattern <u>Understanding of illness and treatments</u>: Resident: *I really don't think I need to be here in this place, it's like I can't take care of things.* Spouse: *He is forgetful at times though he sure is able to tell those stories from long ago.*	**Neurological:** *Alert and oriented to person, needs reminding that is now in the facility, confuses day hour with night hour, calm cooperative, though impatient with length of the assessment, clear speech, hesitant at times, needs questions repeated when he forgets the question, repeats information, forgets he has already answered the question, moves all extremities equally, generalized weakness noted.*
Role–Relationship Pattern <u>Role in family</u> Spouse: *He has always been the one in charge, we have 5 children, 9 grandchildren and a new grandson.* <u>Effect of illness on roles</u> Spouse: *He needs so much help now though he doesn't realize it.*	**Communication Between Family Members:** *Husband and wife communicate well. Wife tends to "fill in the blanks" when spouse seems to lose train of thought or can't find the word.* **Family Visits:** *Wife present with resident, children visit when able due to distance from parents.*
Coping–Stress Tolerance Pattern <u>Stressors</u>: *Being here in the hospital and being put here, I don't want to be here.* <u>Coping methods</u>: *I ignore it—can't do much about that stuff anyway.* <u>Support systems</u>: *Family and church.*	
Value–Belief Pattern <u>Source of hope/strength</u>: *Family and I get a lot of support from Father Joseph at St. Michaels Catholic Church. I sure would like to get back to mass every week.*	**Presence of Religious Articles:** *Bible, rosary.*

Nursing Process: Planning Outcomes

The nurse has identified the key nursing diagnoses for Mr. McClelland. A plan of care now needs to be developed to facilitate the resolution of these identified health issues. It is imperative that the "resolution points" are concisely identified. This "end-point" decision-making process begins the planning phase of the nursing process.

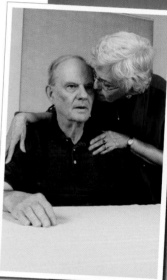

1. Using the ANA *Standards of Practice*, discuss why the planning phase of the nursing process can be described as the road map of patient care.

_____

_____

_____

_____

_____

_____

2. Planning is both an initial and an ongoing process. Discuss this statement within the perspective of Mr. McClelland's admission to your facility.

_____

_____

_____

_____

_____

_____

_____

_____

_____

3. How would the planning of nursing care differ for Mr. McClelland if the admission to the facility was for short-term rehabilitation for reconditioning and strengthening before returning home with his wife? Review the procedure for "Discharging a patient from the healthcare facility" as well as the considerations given to the discharge of an older adult.

_____

_____

_____

_____

_____

_____

_____

_____

_____

_____

_____

_____

_____

_____

4. The comprehensive plan of care for Mr. McClelland needs to address the four different kinds of care. Identify the four kinds of care and give an example that may be applicable to Mr. McClelland's needs.

Type of Care	Examples

5. Describe the common types of standardized care plans. Within the setting of a long-term care facility, give examples that could apply in the provision of nursing care for Mr. McClelland.

Standardized Plan	Examples

6. It is imperative that any standardized nursing care plan be individualized to each patient. Using a standard nursing care plan book, critique the recommended plan of care for "Risk for falls." Consider:
  • Are all the interventions applicable to Mr. McClelland? Explain.

_____

_____

_____

_____

_____

_____

_____

_____

_____

_____

  • Identify factors that need to be addressed to enhance the standard interventions.

_____

_____

_____

_____

_____

7. As the nurse in the facility you also have a nursing student assigned to assist with the care for Mr. McClelland. The student asks, "Why do I have to do so much more than you do on plans of care if I won't be doing that when I graduate?" How would you respond to this question?

_____

_____

_____

_____

_____

_____

8. For each of the five nursing diagnoses previously identified for Mr. McClelland in the nursing diagnosis module, write a broad goal statement.

Nursing Diagnosis	Broad Goal Statement

9. Based on your understanding of the outcome statement (subject, action verb, performance criteria, target time and special conditions) identify a goal statement for each of the five nursing diagnoses identified for Mr. McClelland.

10. Why is it inappropriate to establish a goal for a collaborative problem on the nursing plan of care?

11. Using the Nursing Outcomes Classification (NOC), identify an outcome and two indicators for each of the six identified nursing diagnoses for Mr. McClelland.

Diagnosis	Outcome	Indicators

12. Indicate an appropriate measurement scale for each of the indicators for Mr. McClelland as indicated by his admission data and then the outcome level. Consider: What is the highest level of functioning you can expect to occur after interventions? Discuss your rationales for each.

_____

_____

Outcome	Indicators	Admission	After Interventions

13. Identify a possible learning need for Mr. and Mrs. McClelland. Identify two appropriate objectives to meet this need. Teaching objectives describe what the patient is to learn and the observable behaviors that demonstrate that the learning has been successful. Learning outcomes are categorized as cognitive (the thinking part, knowledge), psychomotor (the doing part, demonstrating skills) or affective (the caring/feeling/attitude part). Assistance for writing these outcomes can be found in the chapter on teaching/learning.

14. Discuss the evaluation process that facilitates your ability to critique and reflect critically about your identified goals and outcomes for Mr. McClelland's plan of care.

Nursing Process: Planning Interventions

The establishment of diagnoses and associated goals for Mr. McClelland now requires nursing interventions, individualized to the patient, to facilitate the meetings of the identified outcomes. Nursing interventions flow from the information provided by the problem (NANDA label) and the etiological factors identified in the nursing diagnostic statement as well as the desired outcomes already identified using the NOC system.

The Nursing Intervention Classification (NIC) provides a standardized comprehensive listing of direct- and indirect-care activities performed by nurses.

List below the six nursing diagnoses (three actual diagnoses, two at risk diagnoses, and one wellness diagnosis) that had been previously identified for Mr. McClelland.

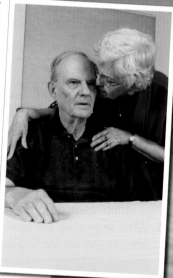

6. Identify three appropriate activities, for one of the NIC interventions under each diagnosis, including at least one from each of the intervention types, if appropriate to the problem status, and provide a rationale for their use in resolving the patient problem.

Outcome	Intervention	Activities	Rationale

Outcome	Intervention	Activities	Rationale

Outcome	Intervention	Activities	Rationale

7. Write appropriate nursing orders that individualize the nine interventions/activities to Mr. McClelland.

DX		
Intervention	**Activities**	**Nursing Orders**

DX		
Intervention	**Activities**	**Nursing Orders**

DX		
Intervention	**Activities**	**Nursing Orders**

8. For each of the following frameworks for prioritizing care, identify the top three nursing orders for each from all of the nursing orders. Discuss how the priorities are similar and how they differ.
- Maslow's Hierarchy of Needs
- Problem urgency
- Future consequences
- Patient preference

Framework	Priorities
Maslow's Hierarchy of Needs	
Problem urgency	
Future consequences	
Patient preference	

_____

_____

_____

_____

_____

_____

_____

Nursing Process: Evaluation

1. After completion of nursing care, the patient's responses are documented in the healthcare record. Why is this important for the evaluation step of the nursing process?

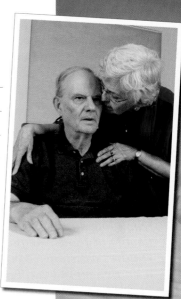

_____

_____

_____

_____

_____

2. Discuss how evaluation is essential to all aspects of the delivery of patient care inclusive of the nursing profession and the healthcare industry itself.

_____

_____

_____

_____

_____

_____

_____

_____

_____

_____

_____

_____

3. Discuss how the three types of evaluation: structure, processes, and outcomes, affect how nursing care may be organized and delivered in a long-term care facility.

_____

_____

_____

_____

_____

_____

_____

_____

_____

_____

The following reassessment data were documented in regard to the plan of care for Mr. McClelland 7 days after admission to the facility:

Awake, alert and oriented to person and place. HOB up 45° Respirations 22 breaths/min and nonlabored, right lung clear and fine crackles noted left base. No wheezing/stridor noted. Denies shortness of breath with activity. Has not required oxygen therapy at night. O₂ sats during sleep 92%–93% on room air. Apical pulse regular at 84 beats/min, no NVD. 1+ edema noted of lower extremities. Abdomen soft with active bowel sounds. Daily BM. Eating 50% of meals, states that food is very tasteless and not pleasant to eat. Needs reminding during mealtimes to eat. Does not care for spices provided to enhance flavors of foods. Requesting salt at every meal. Weight = 139#. Gait unsteady, requires assistance of one person to ambulate to the BR. Voiding qs, noted to need two night voidings. No incidences of incontinence since admission. States, "I can't get any rest in this place." Resting at the scheduled intervals throughout the day. Not calling for assistance when needed, bed/chair alarms on for safety. Wife visits daily, Father Joseph in to visit with resident yesterday. Resident still verbalizing needing to attend mass at his church.

4. Using the reassessment data, write an evaluation statement for each of the identified outcomes for the five diagnoses identified for Mr. McClelland at admission.

Outcome	Evaluative Statement

Outcome	Evaluative statement

5. For each reassessment, determine the status of goal achievement and the evaluative statement using the NOC scale. Give a rationale for the NOC goal indicator.

Outcome	Indicators	Admission Data	Goal	Status of Goal Achievement

6. For unmet or partially met goals, relate the outcomes to the interventions/activities determined in the planning intervention phase of the nursing process. What concerns should be addressed and are there needed modifications to the plan of care? Consider each step of the nursing process in this review and revision of the plan of care.

Evaluative Statement	Unmet/Partially Unmet Goals	Interventions/ Activities	Needed Modification

Evaluative Statement	Unmet/Partially Unmet Goals	Interventions/ Activities	Needed Modification

(Continued)

Evaluative Statement	Unmet/Partially Unmet Goals	Interventions/ Activities	Needed Modification

Nursing Process: Implementation

The implementation phase of the nursing process is the doing, delegating, and documenting phase. It is, in essence, the nursing care provided to a patient to meet the identified health status. Implementation of Mr. McClelland's plan of care requires the nurse to have a self-awareness of his or her own knowledge and abilities in regard to the intervention activities and an ability to organize the activities to maximize resources. Use your textbook/procedure guides to help you understand the different activities done with the patient.

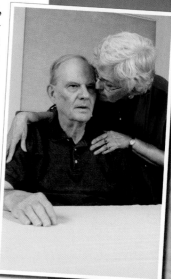

1. List the nine nursing activities previously identified for Mr. McClelland's nursing diagnoses. As a nursing student, identify the knowledge/skills needed to complete each activity. Are you ready/qualified to implement care? Do any of the activities have an inherent safety risk (to you or the patient) when implementing that nursing order?

Intervention	Nursing Orders	Knowledge/Skills

Intervention	Nursing Orders	Knowledge/Skills

Intervention	Nursing Orders	Knowledge/Skills

Intervention	Nursing Orders	Knowledge/Skills

Intervention	Nursing Orders	Knowledge/Skills

2. In organizing care for Mr. McClelland, discuss which activities can be grouped together to best use your time and resources when you are providing care.

_____

_____

_____

_____

_____

_____

_____

_____

_____

_____

3. In the table provided, indicate the activities that directly affect Mr. McClelland. These are activities that are done to or with the patient.

4. Write a _short_ statement for each of these activities that represents how the nurse would explain what is to be done and what Mr. McClelland can expect to feel during each activity.

Activity	Short Description

Activity	Short Description

(Continued)

9. After the completion of nursing care, it is necessary to document the nursing activity and the patient's response. Why is this documentation a critical link in the healthcare delivery system? Consider the aspects of collaboration and coordination of services.

Nursing Theory

Regardless of practice setting, nursing theory is the foundational structure that supports full-spectrum nursing. Theory helps organize how nurses think and facilitate the development of new ideas as well as insights into the work of nursing practice.

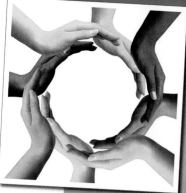

1. Describe the basic components of a nursing theory as you see it supporting the premises of care and comfort within the practice of nursing. Consider:
   • What are your assumptions about care and comfort?

   _____

   _____

   _____

   _____

   • What is this phenomenon of nursing and care?

   _____

   _____

   _____

   _____

   _____

   _____

   _____

   _____

   _____

   _____

• What are the basic concepts related to care and comfort?

_____

_____

_____

_____

_____

_____

_____

_____

_____

• How do you define care and comfort?

_____

_____

_____

_____

_____

_____

_____

_____

_____

_____

_____

_____

_____

_____

Consider the 72-year-old patient who has total left-sided paralysis from a stroke. She is unable to move or feel the left side of her body and has some difficulty swallowing her food and liquids. Before the stroke, she was very active in her community and church and independent in all activities of daily living. The patient is left-handed. For this situation, the patient has no problems with communication. Care for this patient, based in nursing theory, requires logical reasoning to best develop and provide optimal care for her.

2. Why is this ability to be able to reason logically so vital to full-spectrum nursing?

_____

_____

_____

_____

3. For this patient, give an example of inductive reasoning and deductive reasoning when assessing her ability to eat her meal tray.

_____

_____

_____

_____

_____

_____

4. Choose one of the following nurse theorists:
- Virginia Henderson
- Faye Abdellah

Discuss how the theory can be applied to guide nursing practice and support meeting the basic care and comfort needs of this patient. In basic care and comfort, the nurse provides comfort and assistance in the performance of activities of daily living (NCS-BON, 2010, pp. 28–30).
https://www.ncsbn.org/2010_NCLEX_RN_Detailed_Test_Plan_Candidate.pdf

_____

_____

_____

_____

_____

_____

_____

_____

_____

_____

_____

5. How is each of the following theories from other disciplines important to nursing's scientific knowledge base when you are considering care for this patient?
- Maslow's Hierarchy of Human Needs

_____

_____

_____

_____

_____

_____

- Selye's Stress & Adaptation Theory

_____

_____

_____

_____

- Erickson's Psychosocial Developmental Theory

_____

_____

_____

Research

After 2 weeks in the first clinical rotation the student noted that the residents of the dementia unit were often very sad and withdrawn. He also noted that one of the nursing assistants often talked to the residents about their childhood memories, tales of growing up and other life stories. This noticeably lessened the residents' sadness and improved their well-being. The student wondered, "Is this a good way to help with these behaviors rather than just giving them their medications [such as selective serotonin reuptake inhibitors (SSRIs)]?"

Interventions for nursing care should be grounded in evidence-based practice. "Evidence-based practice is a problem-solving approach to the delivery of health care that integrates the best evidence from studies and patient care data with clinician expertise and patient preferences and values" (Fineout-Overholt, Melnyk, Stillway, & Williamson, 2010, p. 58).

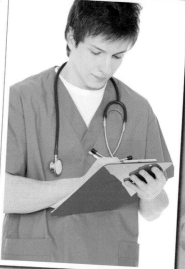

1. Based on your educational preparation, what would be your role in a research project that looked at the use of reminiscence therapy for persons with dementia?

_____

_____

_____

_____

_____

_____

_____

_____

_____

2. Using your understanding of quantitative vs. qualitative research, how could you use each type to help you answer your clinical question?

_____

_____

_____

_____

_____

_____

_____

_____

_____

   After a discussion with the nursing instructor, the student was encouraged to find information that addressed the intervention of reminiscence therapy. With this as your focus, address each one of the following steps of the research process.

3. Formulate a searchable research question using the PICO acronym.

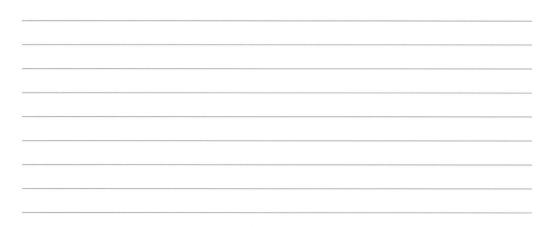

P	Patient Population or Problem	
I	Intervention/treatment/cause/factor	
C	Comparison intervention	
O	Outcome	

_____

_____

_____

4. Search the literature:

 • What evidence supports the use of reminiscence therapy to improve mood and behavior? (key words: reminiscence therapy, dementia, well-being, cognitive impairment)

 • Find at least five citations of articles that appear to address the research topic.

Citations

5. Choose one of the articles you found in your search and decide if it is worthy enough to use as a basis for your research. Discuss the article from the framework of reading analytically:

Citations	
What is the article about as a whole? Describe the theme of the article.	
What are the main ideas, claims, and arguments about the subject?	
Does it seem "legitimate"? Consider the authors' credentials, purpose, problem statement, definition of terms, setting/population, and the findings and conclusions. Are there limitations to the findings?	

(Continued)

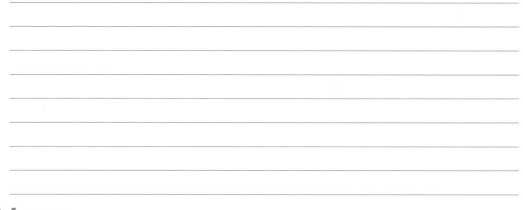

6. Overall, are the results of this article significant to the improvement of the patient care issue that was identified? What might be some barriers to its use in the facility?

_____

_____

_____

_____

_____

_____

_____

_____

_____

_____

_____

References

Fineout-Overholt, E., Melnyk, B.M., Stillway, S. B., & Williamson, K.M. (2010). Evidence-based practice step by step: Asking the clinical question: A key step in evidence-based practice. *American Journal of Nursing, 110*(3): 58–61.

Factors Affecting Health

Growth and Development

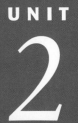

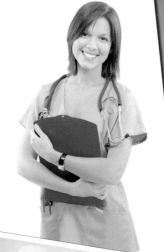

During her community nursing rotation, nursing student Elise Braun is assigned to work with a parish nurse. "Parish nurses are licensed, registered nurses who practice holistic health for self, individuals, and the community using nursing knowledge combined with spiritual care. They function as members of the pastoral team in a variety of religious faiths, cultures, and countries. The focus of their work is on the intentional care of the spirit, assisting the members of the faith community to maintain and/or regain wholeness in body, mind, and spirit" (International Parish Nurse Resource Center, 2012).

http://www.parishnurses.org/WhatisaParishNurseFaith CommunityNurse_299.aspx Retrieved June 15, 2012

The nurse has scheduled sessions today to meet with various groups within the parish. The first group is composed of first-time mothers and is set up for them to discuss concerns regarding their children ages 6 months through 12 months.

1. When meeting with the mothers' group, they voice concern that their children are all "so different" in their development. One member asks, "Why aren't they all pretty much the same?"

Another mother is concerned that there is "something wrong." What should be your first response?

_____

_____

2. Discuss the expected physical development for children between 6 months and 12 months.

_____

_____

_____

_____

_____

_____

_____

_____

_____

_____

3. For a new mother, every stage of her child's development brings both delight and worries. How would you respond to the mother who asks, "What are the major health issues I need to be aware of for my infant?"

_____

_____

_____

_____

_____

_____

_____

_____

_____

_____

_____

_____

_____

_____

_____

_____

_____

_____

_____

_____

The next meeting is with the youth pastor. He has requested a session for a small group of children who will be middle school students in the new school year. They will be attending the summer youth camp at the church, and the youth pastor would like the nurse to discuss issues inherent to this new phase of their lives.

4. The parish nurse wants to develop an awareness program of the common health problems encountered by this age group. Discuss the issues that need to be addressed.

_____

5. Which issue would be most appropriate as the *initial* session with this age group? Give a rationale for your choice.

6. Describe how the major psychological tasks (Erickson) of adolescence need to be incorporated into the teaching/learning strategies to facilitate the success of this program.

_____

_____

_____

_____

_____

_____

_____

_____

_____

_____

_____

_____

_____

_____

_____

The last session is the weekly meeting of the "seasoned citizen" group. They meet to discuss issues pertinent to healthy independent living for older members and always like "their nurse" to attend.

7. The parish nurse comments to you, "Just getting together is one of the best strategies I could recommend to this group." What is the implication of this statement in regard to the elderly and their health status?

_____

_____

_____

_____

8. A goal of health promotion for this age group is maintenance of an exercise program. Discuss the activities appropriate to this parish nursing program at the church.

_____

_____

_____

_____

_____

_____

_____

_____

_____

_____

_____

_____

_____

_____

_____

_____

_____

_____

_____

_____

_____

_____

_____

_____

_____

_____

_____

_____

_____

_____

_____

9. The nurse tells you, "I always do a modified assessment on all the attendees when I visit their group each month." Discuss the physical assessments that can easily be done in this setting.

_____

_____

_____

10. Discuss how an understanding and integration of Erickson's developmental theory and the task stage for this group are vital to the development of strategies that support holistic care of this population.

Health and Illness

Mrs. Watson, an 81-year-old, is scheduled to be admitted to your rehabilitation center from the hospital for short-term rehabilitation. She is part of a care continuum program for patients who have undergone hip replacement surgery. The program philosophy recognizes that each patient experiences the illness differently and strives to develop and implement an individualized plan of care that will enhance recovery and an overall sense of wellness.

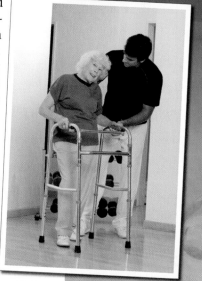

On admission Mrs. Watson tells the nurse, "I am very nervous about being here. So much is at stake—if I don't do well they won't let me go home by myself. I was so used to taking care of myself before I fell and broke my hip. This has been hard. Except for some joint stiffness in the morning I really don't have anything wrong with me and I am proud of that! I've never had to take any regular medications. I've always been a can-do person and going all the time; active in my church, volunteer at the senior center to help with the elderly folks and help watch my great-grandbaby who just turned 1—he is a handful! Now I feel like I can't take care of myself anymore and I am afraid this will happen again. It has been hard to deal with the pain and discomfort of both the injury and the process of getting well. I've never thought of myself as 'old and feeble' until now and I don't like it. Only old people use walkers! I've got so much I still want to do!"

1. Discuss the factors that Mrs. Watson is facing that are considered to have disrupted her health.

Factor	Disrupted Factors Applicable to Mrs. Watson

2. What stage of illness behavior is she exhibiting at admission?

Stages of Illness Behavior	Presentation

3. For each of the behaviors essential to communicating genuine care, concern, and sensitivity, give an example of how you would use these in your interaction with Mrs. Watson.

Psychosocial Health and Illness

A patient's ability to respond to illness is influenced not only by the physical illness itself but also by the patient's psychosocial health, inclusive of psychological and social factors.

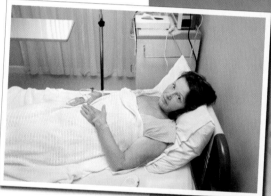

You are caring for two patients on the burn unit. They are in the intermediate phase of burn recovery, meaning that they have survived their injuries, are physiologically stable, and moving slowly toward recovery.

- Mrs. Castile, a 79-year-old burned in a mobile home fire. Burns to legs, and inhalation injury (lungs)
- Ms. Locklear, a 23-year-old injured and burned in a motor vehicle accident. Burns to chest, abdomen, right arm and right leg, and crush injury resulting in amputation of the right foot.

1. After reading each woman's abbreviated health history, identify three important psychosocial influences for each patient that may help or hinder her recovery.

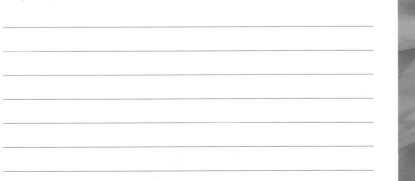

_____

_____

_____

_____

_____

Burn injury and the sequelae of recovery constitute a major assault on the patient's self-concept and self-esteem. Self-concept is affected by many factors inclusive of gender, developmental level, family and peer relationships and internal influences.

2. Discuss these factors and how you think they will influence each of the patient's self-concept in light of her present health crisis?

Factors	Mrs. Castile	Ms. Locklear
Gender		
Developmental level		
Relationships		
Internal influences		

3. Discuss the components of self-concept and how each patient may respond to the changes secondary to her burn injuries.

Component	Mrs. Castile	Ms. Locklear

Two psychosocial illnesses that nurses will commonly deal with in any practice setting are anxiety and depression. This is especially true when patients are experiencing a major health crisis as every level of need is threatened by the situation.

4. For each patient you are caring for, identify potential threats to her basic needs (Maslow) that can be anxiety producing. Keep in mind that anxiety is a vague emotional response to a known or an unknown threat; therefore, you can be somewhat creative in thinking about potential threats.

Level of Maslow	Mrs. Castile	Ms. Locklear
Physiological		
Safety/security		
Love/belonging		
Esteem		
Self-actualization		

5. After one particularly difficult physical therapy session, Ms. Locklear tells you, "I never do anything right in PT and no matter what I do in there things are never going to change how I look or get me back to where I was before the accident." You identify a diagnosis of Disturbed Body Image[†] with the NOC outcome of Body Image. What would be appropriate individualized outcomes for Ms. Locklear in light of her injuries?

_____

_____

_____

_____

_____

_____

6. Develop individualized nursing actions for the NIC intervention Body Image Enhancement.

_____

_____

_____

_____

7. Mrs. Castile is at a higher risk for depression as it is a common emotional disorder of older adults. What data in her health history indicate a risk for depression?

_____

_____

_____

[†]© 2012 NANDA International

_____

_____

_____

8. The physical therapist returns Mrs. Castile from therapy and tells you, "I think all this happening to her has affected her mental state—this change in location and major health crisis sure has changed her. I think it has triggered an onset of dementia. She says she cannot complete anything because she is 'totally exhausted all the time.' She used to enjoy the challenge of therapy. She seems confused at times and she doesn't want to follow her therapy orders. She told me she 'just wants to be left alone and I wish I were dead.' She is just so sad now. I think she needs some medication for early onset dementia—can you talk to the primary care provider about this?" Which data indicate that Mrs. Castile may need follow-up for depression?

_____

_____

_____

_____

_____

_____

_____

_____

9. Is Mrs. Castile at risk for suicide? Why or why not?

_____

_____

10. Discuss the interventions for suicide prevention and how they can be implemented within the constraints of both Mrs. Castile's environment and her specific situation.

_____

_____

_____

_____

Patient: Mrs. Castile	**Ethnic Origin:** American	**Religion:** Christian/Roman Catholic
Current Age: 79 years old	**Marital Status:** Widow	**Education:** 8th grade
Gender: Female	**Culture:** Italian American	**Insurance:** Medicare/Medicaid
Race: Caucasian		

Source of History
Mrs. Castile is a reliable source of history. She was alert and oriented x3.

Reason for Seeking Care
"I am here to get better from my burns."

History of Present Illness
Patient is 79-year-old female burned in a mobile home fire. Burns to legs and inhalation injury (lungs). Required grafting to leg burns, still receiving oxygen therapy to maintain oxygen saturation > 92% on 2L/min and will need this upon discharge due to lung damage and subsequent pulmonary compromise.

PAST HEALTH
Accidents or Injuries
Reports no prior accidents or injuries.

Serious or Chronic Illnesses
Reports a history of "palpitations" and atrial fibrillation. Has been told she has "heart problems" but denies heart attack, congestive heart failure, hypertension, and diabetes.

Hospitalizations
Reports hospitalization for irregular heartbeats at age 67, "I was feeling so woozy headed when my heart acted up." They did a lot of tests but all they said was I had an irregular rhythm and gave me medications. I have done ok since then.

Operations
Skin grafting to lower legs with this admission. Appendectomy "as a child—I think I might have been six or seven at the time. I don't remember having any trouble from it."

Allergies
Denies any allergies.

Current Medications
Reports taking Lanoxin 0.125 mg daily, Coumadin 2 mg M-W-F, 1 mg T-R-Sat-Sun, multivitamin daily, and Miralax 17g daily in 8 oz juice. PRN medications include Percocet one-two tabs q4h for moderate pain, Tylenol 650 mg q4h (not to exceed 4 grams in 24 hrs) for mild pain.

REVIEW OF SYSTEMS
General Overall Health State
Height: 5'3". Weight: 147 lb. Prior to this accident I was doing ok with getting around and doing the things I needed to do. "Now I don't know what will become of me."

FUNCTIONAL ASSESSMENT
Self-esteem, Self-Concept
She identifies herself as hardworking, dependable, and caring. Reports that she feels she is able to take care of herself.

Health Practices and Beliefs
Reports going to the doctor when she feels like she is getting sick or notices a problem. Reports she tries to follow the doctor's advice and take her meds as needed.

Recreation, Pets, and Hobbies
Reports three cats; Chloe (10 years old), Bear (2 years old), and Lilly (6 months old). Patient reports that she loved to spend time with her pets. Pets lost in fire event.

Interpersonal Relationships/Resources
Patient describes her role in the family as a grandmother. Patients reports she lost her son to cancer last month and he was her main support. "I don't see as much of my grandchildren as I would like now."

Spiritual Resources
Reports attending church daily for mass. Reports a very strong belief in God and states "He will help me through this." Denies having any specific religious practices that should be incorporated into the plan of care.

Coping and Stress Management
Reports feeling overwhelmed with being in the burn unit. Reports unable to sleep and feeling hopeless about ever getting to go home.

Cultural Practices
Denies any cultural influences on her health practices. Does not participate in any cultural practices or events regularly.

Socioeconomic Status
Reports having medical insurance. Reports that she has struggled with finances "it's hard to live on social security."

Patient: Ms. Locklear
Current Age: 23 years old
Gender: Female
Race: Native American

Ethnic Origin: American
Marital Status: Single
Culture: Native American

Religion: Christian
Education: College graduate/BS degree
Insurance: Blue Cross/Blue Shield

Source of History
Ms. Locklear is a reliable source of history. She was alert and oriented x3.

Reason for Seeking Care
"I was brought to the burn unit after my car wreck—I still am not sure what happened it happened so fast!" I know I am in the intermediate unit to get me back to my normal self.

History of Present Illness
Patient is 23 years old, single, injured and burned in a motor vehicle accident. Burns to chest, abdomen, right arm and right leg, crush injury resulting in amputation of the right foot, spent 4 weeks in the ICU before transfer to intermediate unit.

PAST HEALTH
Accidents or Injuries
Reports a four wheeler accident at age 15. Patient flipped the four wheeler in a ditch. Did not suffer any injuries. Reports a car accident at age 21. Vehicle rolled two and a half times and patient was taken to Regional Medical Center, by ambulance, for evaluation. Patient suffered only minor injuries (scratches and bruising).

Serious or Chronic Illnesses
Denies any heart diseases, hypertension, diabetes, cancer, or seizures.

Hospitalizations
Reports hospitalization for croup at 18 months old, denies any respiratory issues related to incident.

Operations
Multiple skin grafts to chest, abdomen, and right leg with this admission.

Allergies
Denies any allergies.

Current Medications
Celexa 10 mg tablet daily. PRN medications include Percocet one-two tabs q4h for moderate pain, Tylenol 650 mg q4h (not to exceed 4 grams in 24 hrs) for mild pain.

REVIEW OF SYSTEMS
General Overall Health State
Height: 5'7½". Weight: 127 lb. Prior to this accident no health issues.

FUNCTIONAL ASSESSMENT
Self-esteem, Self-Concept
Reports "feels ok" about herself. Reports, "I can't seem to get a break sometimes. I seem to have bad karma—everything happens to me and its outside of my control." Reports that she is concerned about her appearance with scarring from the burns and grafts, "I look so ugly." Reports she does not handle stress well, "I've always been on something to help with my stress." She considers herself shy before she gets to know someone.

Health Practices and Beliefs
Patient expresses importance of having annual checkups and exams. Reports "I try to take care of myself." Reports going to the doctor when she feels like she is getting sick or notices a problem.

Recreation, Pets, and Hobbies
Reports she likes to read and was training for a 5K run with a group from work prior to the accident. Denies having pets.

Interpersonal Relationships/Resources
Patient describes her role in the family as a daughter, granddaughter, and sister. Patient names her mother as her main support system.

Spiritual Resources
Reports attending church "once in a while" when mother insists that she go. Denies having any specific religious practices that should be incorporated into the plan of care.

Coping and Stress Management
Reports having stress due to pressures at work. Reports has always been "stressed" and tends to struggle with feeling down at times. Reports not dealing well with the burns, states, "I am so ugly now—I just can't deal with it all."

Cultural Practices
Denies any cultural influences on her health practices. Does not participate in any cultural practices or events regularly.

Socioeconomic Status
Reports having medical insurance, vision insurance, and dental through her job. Reports she was "doing ok" financially before the accident.

Family

Family is described as two or more individuals who provide physical, emotional, economic, or spiritual support while maintaining involvement in one another's lives. Families come in many forms, living arrangements, and emotional connections.

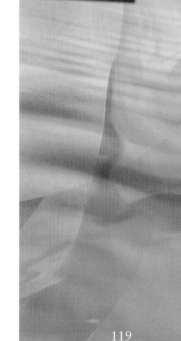

You are the hospice nurse assigned to an elderly couple referred to your agency by their primary care provider. The husband has end-stage cardiac disease. He is adamant about staying in his own home and refuses placement in a long-term care facility as well as having any person coming into the home to provide personal care. The spouse is the primary caregiver and assumes responsibility for all his care. They have five children, three sons and two daughters, all of whom live out of state. The daughters try to schedule visits so that one of them visits at least once a month entailing drives of 6 and 8 hours, respectively. They speak with you regularly, with their parents' permission, to stay engaged in the plan of care for their father. The sons have voiced that care of the parents is "the girls' job," although the sons are now demanding placement for their father. They have commented, "The nursing home will make it easier on everyone if someone else has the responsibility for all the care that is needed. That is what those places are for anyway; why make it so hard on Mom? Dad is being selfish." The sons' lack of support for the father's wishes has created conflict within the family.

The spouse has verbalized "I should be able to take care of everything; I am a retired nurse so I know what needs to be done." You note that she is continuously preoccupied with the care routine to the extent that she lacks the time to meet her own personal and social needs. She confides in you that she really misses the ability to go to daily mass and attend her weekly exercise class at the health center. She is afraid to leave her husband alone. She admits to having difficulty sleeping, saying, "What if I don't hear him call me at night when he needs something?" In addition she worries that she won't always be able to provide all his care and she knows that bringing in outside help or placing him in a long-term care facility is not an option because that is

5. Assess the family's communication pattern and the family's coping processes.

_____

_____

_____

_____

_____

_____

_____

_____

_____

_____

_____

_____

6. After analyzing the data gathered from the family members regarding the situation, you identify a diagnosis of Family Processes, Interrupted.[†] What cues indicated the applicability of this diagnostic label for this family? Use the characteristics of a healthy family to determine deviation from norms.

Characteristics of a Healthy Family	Analysis/Cues of Family Family Processes, Interrupted
State of family well-being	
Sense of belonging and connectedness	
Clear boundaries between family members	
Sense of trust and respect	
Honesty and freedom of expression	
Time together; sharing rituals	
Relaxed body language	
Flexibility/adaptability and ability to deal with stress	
Commitment	
Spiritual well-being	
Respect for privacy	
Balance of giving and receiving	
Positive, effective communication	
Accountability	
Appreciation/affection for each other	
Responding to needs and interests of all members	
Health promoting lifestyle of individual members	

7. In addition you identify a diagnosis of Caregiver Role Strain.† What are the defining characteristics present in this care situation that validates this diagnosis?

_____

_____

_____

_____

_____

_____

_____

_____

_____

_____

_____

_____

_____

_____

8. Identify an NOC outcome for each of these diagnoses as well as individualized outcomes specifically to this particular family situation.

Diagnosis†	NOC	Individualized Outcomes
Family Processes, Interrupted		
Caregiver Role Strain		

†© 2012 NANDA International

9. Identify two NIC interventions for each outcome and individualize them to this particular family situation.

Diagnosis[†]	NOC Outcome	NIC Interventions	Individualized to Family
Family Processes Interrupted			
Caregiver Role Strain			

10. Review one of the following resources available for caregivers and healthcare professionals and discuss how the information from the site is beneficial to both you as the nurse and your assigned family.
- http://www.caregiving.com—Family Caregiving
- http://www.caregiver.org—Family Caregiver Alliance
- http://www.nfcacares.org—National Family Caregiving Association

Culture
and Ethnicity

Mia Yaj is a patient on your postpartum unit. She gave birth to a baby boy 7 hours ago. Her husband and her grandmother have been with her throughout the entire birth experience. Although she is a college graduate, Ms. Yaj feels pressured to adhere to her culture's traditional ways of healing in the postpartum period to appease family expectations. Despite her desire to avoid any medications, she has had several doses of a medication for pain control. She lists her culture and that of her family as Hmong. The grandmother immigrated to

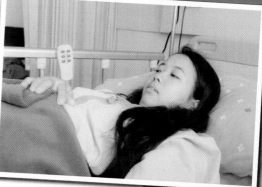

the United States from Laos in 1977 along with her four children, one of whom is the patient's mother. The grandmother does not speak/understand English well and Ms. Yaj normally acts as her interpreter. Ms. Yaj was born and raised in the United States. Her husband is also of the Hmong culture, having immigrated with his parents as an infant. He too is a college graduate. He is supportive of his wife's adherence to the postpartum healing rituals.

1. How are the cultural concepts of socialization, acculturation, and assimilation portrayed by this family system?

_____

_____

_____

_____

_____

_____

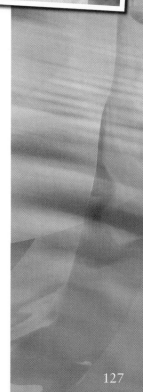

_____

_____

_____

_____

_____

_____

_____

_____

_____

_____

_____

_____

_____

_____

2. Discuss any subcultural characteristics of this couple that make them different from the family's main Hmong culture.

_____

_____

_____

_____

_____

3. How would you designate their ethnicity and race on the mother's electronic health record?

_____

_____

4. How could each of the following culture specifics influence the plan of care for Ms. Yaj?

_____

_____

_____

_____

_____

_____

_____

a. Communication:

_____

_____

_____

_____

_____

_____

b. Space:

_____

_____

c. Time orientation:

_____

_____

_____

_____

_____

d. Social organization:

_____

_____

_____

   This family system's healthcare model is a combination of the indigenous healthcare system and the professional healthcare system. The couple chose to deliver the baby at the hospital with the use of a certified nurse midwife in attendance. The child will not be circumcised. The new mother will follow the Hmong birth recuperation process of restricting her diet to only chicken/white rice, warm water, and tea made with loose tea for 30 days after delivery. No other foods or cold drinks are allowed during this time. A regular diet will be resumed after this 30-day period. The grandmother will be the primary support/caregiver during this period. It is vital for you, as the nurse, to practice culturally competent care for optimal recovery and functioning of this family unit.

5. How does your cultural sensitivity and competence affect the development and delivery of patient care for this family?

_____

_____

_____

Spirituality

While working with her assigned resident, Mrs. Edna Harrison, in the long-term care facility, Bethany Fisher, a first-year nursing student, is suddenly asked by the resident, "Do you believe in God?" Before she can answer the resident adds, "I've lost my ability to talk to God. It feels like God has forgotten us in this place. There is so much pain and suffering that just shouldn't be." Bethany recognizes that Mrs. Harrison is reaching out regarding spiritual issues in her life.

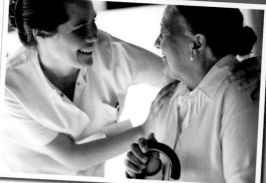

1. Bethany knows very little about the resident's religious background or practices. Therefore, what should her first response be to these statements?

_____

_____

_____

_____

2. Discuss the barriers to spiritual care that may impede Bethany's ability to meet the spiritual needs of this resident.

_____

_____

_____

_____

_____

_____

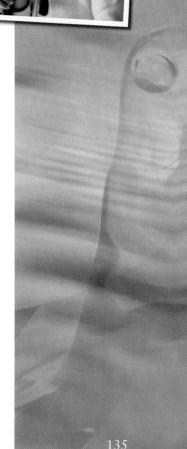

With guidance, Bethany completes a spiritual assessment using the HOPE tool. The assessment data include the following:

H: Sources of hope, meaning, comfort, strength, peace, love, and connection

My religious beliefs have always been a source of comfort and strength when dealing with my ups and downs but now it doesn't seem to sustain me or even make sense. I have lost my belief, I think, as I have watched so many of us sicken, suffer, and die. I have always read my Bible, prayed, and attended services, but even those have gone by the wayside. They used to give me such strength to handle things—the hardest being when my husband and son both died in the same year and even when I first moved into the home.

O: Organized religion

I've always been active in the Presbyterian Church even when my husband was so sick. It was important to me to have that connection with other people as well as with my God. I felt closest to God when I was attending services. I am still a member and on occasion some of my friends do visit me here. The minister visits too but not as often as I need right now. I enjoy seeing them and it does help me feel better at times.

P: Personal spirituality/practices

I used to believe in God; well . . . I think I still do—he just seems to be absent in the life around here—does that make sense? I have always enjoyed my prayer time and reading my Bible. I like listening to hymns too but now they seem so mournful. I miss the joy.

E: Effects on medical care and end-of-life issues

Being here has changed how often I can participate in church activities. Being here has made me realize how futile so much of what we believe will help. Why

does there have to be so much suffering when you are sick or when you need help with daily activities like I do? Sometimes it seems that what they want me to do as far as healthcare seems to be at odds with what I believe is the will of God . . . which seems wrong somehow. For instance, they have this feeding tube in my stomach because I haven't been able to eat safely since I had my stroke. Maybe I am not supposed to be still alive—maybe not being able to eat was a sign it was my time? I just don't know what the answers are and I find it difficult to handle these days.

3. Bethany identifies the issue of Spiritual distress.[†] Identify the validating defining characteristics of this diagnosis from the initial interaction as well as the assessment data.

Defining Characteristics	Patient Data

4. As etiological factors, what nursing diagnoses could also apply to this situation? Identify the defining characteristics present in the initial interaction and the assessment data that support these diagnoses.

Nursing Diagnostic Label	Defining Characteristics	Patient Data

5. For the nursing diagnosis Spiritual Distress,[†] identify the two NOC standardized outcomes most applicable to Mrs. Harrison's problem and individualize the outcome statements to reflect her needs.

_____

_____

_____

_____

_____

_____

_____

_____

_____

_____

_____

_____

_____

_____

_____

6. Bethany chooses the NIC interventions active listening and spiritual support. Individualize the interventions to this resident's protestant religion. How would the interventions change in light of the following differing religions?
a. Protestantism (Mrs. Harrison)
b. Judaism
c. Seventh-Day Adventism
d. Islam
e. Buddhism
f. Native American religions

Religion	Interventions Active Listening Spiritual Support	
Protestantism (Mrs. Harrison)		

	Modifications (if needed) Active Listening Spiritual Support	
Judaism		
Seventh-Day Adventism		

(Continued)

	Modifications (if needed) Active Listening Spiritual Support	
Islam		
Buddhism		
Native American religions		

7. Mrs. Harrison asks Bethany to pray for her. What further information does Bethany need from the resident to best meet this request?

8. Compose a prayer that includes the information that Bethany has received from Mrs. Harrison.

Loss, Grief, and Dying

You are the hospice nurse at a residential hospice house caring for Mrs. Shona Williams, a 41-year-old African American female, who has been diagnosed with Stage IV breast cancer with metastasis to the bone. She has undergone surgery and chemotherapy but neither has stopped the progression of the disease and she is terminally ill. She is expressing the following sentiments as she deals with the outcomes of her disease:

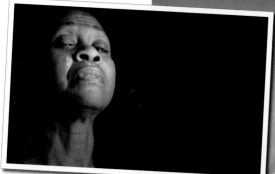

- *I feel I've lost all that makes me a woman.*
- *Sometimes I get so angry about this I cry out in frustration— I know I take it out on my daughters. . . They are so young, only 12 and 17 years old and it is unfair to them.*
- *I will never get to see my daughters go to college, get married, or have my grandchildren; I've lost the best years of my life that were yet to come.*
- *I am trying to figure out why this has happened to me— I've always been a good person.*
- *Why did God do this to me? To my family?*
- *My husband and children refuse to discuss plans of a future without me—I worry about them dealing with all this.*
- *I don't want to suffer at the end—please don't let me. How do I keep the system from prolonging my agony and that of my family?*

1. Describe the categories of loss that are demonstrated by Mrs. Williams's statements.

_____

_____

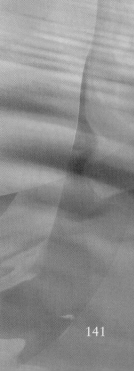

_____

_____

_____

_____

_____

_____

_____

_____

_____

_____

_____

_____

2. The diagnostic label Grieving[†] is identified for the patient. Write a three-part nursing diagnostic statement that reflects the patient's response to this situation.

_____

_____

_____

_____

3. What other nursing diagnoses can be identified for this patient? Give the supporting data for each.

Diagnosis	Rationale/Patient Data Supporting Dx

4. Discuss how hospice care is an integral part of meeting the needs identified in the nursing diagnoses listed for the patient.

_____

_____

_____

_____

_____

_____

_____

_____

_____

_____

_____

_____

_____

_____

_____

5. As the hospice nurse, how would you explain the need for advance directives and a DNAR order with this family system?

_____

_____

_____

_____

_____

_____

_____

_____

_____

_____

_____

_____

_____

_____

_____

6. During the last days of her life, Mrs. Williams becomes unresponsive. She is on pain medications to keep her comfortable, and her family has been with her most of the time. How can you best meet the needs of the family at this time?

_____

_____

_____

_____

_____

_____

_____

7. Upon the death of Mrs. Williams, what should you do to support the family?

_____

_____

_____

_____

8. Discuss the delegation instructions you should give to the nursing assistant assigned to complete Mrs. Williams's postmortem care.

_____

_____

_____

_____

_____

_____

9. The nursing assistant comes to you and states, "I can't get the patient's mouth to stay closed. What should I do?" How would you respond?

_____

_____

_____

With the death of Mrs. Williams, the focus of nursing care shifts to care of the family and their needs in regard to their grieving the loss of wife/mother.

10. Discuss how the factors affecting grief as well as the developmental stage may affect the grieving process for Mr. Williams and each of his daughters.

11. A diagnosis of Grieving[†] related to loss of significant other as evidenced by psychological distress and despair is identified. An NOC outcome of Family Resiliency is established with the family. Identify appropriate NIC interventions and individualize them to this family situation within the parameters of developmental and life needs.

_____

_____

_____

_____

_____

_____

_____

_____

_____

_____

_____

_____

_____

_____

_____

_____

_____

_____

_____

12. As the healthcare provider, you too experience a sense of loss. How can you best take care of yourself? How could this experience help or hinder your role as a hospice nurse?

_____

_____

_____

_____

_____

_____

_____

_____

UNIT

Essential Nursing Interventions

3

Documenting and Reporting

Beginning her clinical preparation the evening before, this morning Melanie Lindler finds she has been assigned to care for a 68-year-old male with a medical diagnosis of diabetic ketoacidosis and dehydration. She will be caring for him on his second hospital day.

1. What type of information can Melanie find in each of the following documentation forms? Why is that information vital to her preparation for care of her assigned client?
- Nursing admission data form:

_____

_____

_____

_____

- Graphic record:

_____

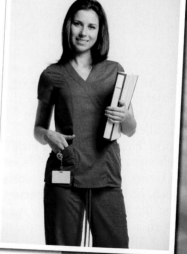

- Intake & output:

_____

_____

- Medication Administration Record:

_____

_____

_____

_____

_____

_____

_____

_____

_____

_____

_____

_____

_____

_____

_____

_____

_____

At 0700 the morning of her clinical day she and her co-assigned RN receive the following report from the off-going shift RN:

Mr. Howard Devon in 3115 is a 68-year-old male admitted yesterday with DKA. He is allergic to codeine. He is HOH. His admitting glucose was 758 with severe dehydration. He is AAO × 2, a little confused about where he is at but he's been through so many changes in the last 24 hours. He reorients easily. He has O_2 on at 2 L/min via NC, O_2 sats running 90–91, lungs are clear, he gets breathing treatments every 6 hours and prn, he has COPD. Heart rate irregular in the 70s, I think they said he has a-fib—he is on dig for that. Skin is warm and dry, still got pretty bad skin turgor, abdomen soft with active bowel sounds, no bowel movement since admission. His FBS this morning was 287 and he received coverage with 6 units of Novalog. Make sure he eats a good breakfast, will you? He has NS at 125 mL/hr into his right hand, it's a #20, site looks good. The pump has beeped a lot—I think it is positional and I told him to keep it up on a pillow. He is voiding well. He has a UTI, which is probably what put him into DKA this time. He needs help getting to the bathroom because of the pump and he has a sore foot. We have been assisting him to use the urinal. He is on Fall Precautions. He has an ulcer on his right foot that the wound team has been treating on an outpatient basis. Right now we are just doing wet to moist dressing changes bid, I changed the dressing around 2100. There is a surgical consult for it, it looks pretty bad and he might lose part of that foot. He is on IV antibiotics too. He gets one Percocet for the foot pain every 6 hours, last one was at 0120 so he is probably due for another. He rates his pain at a 10 before his meds and a 6–7 afterward. He might need something besides the Percocet. He had a pretty good night except for the pump, any questions?

2. There is a lot of information received on this patient in the abbreviated language of nursing. Using your resources, interpret the terms used in this report.

3. Identify the descriptors that inadequately present patient status and replace them with professional or more complete terms. When reporting information it is important to give objective (fact-based) descriptors rather than subjective (opinion: good, bad, ok) descriptors. You may need to seek assistance in understanding all the information regarding this patient to correctly document his status.

■ Mr. Howard Devon in 3115 is a 68-year-old male admitted yesterday with DKA. He is allergic to codeine. He is HOH. His admitting glucose was 758 with severe dehydration. He is AAO × 2, little confused about where he is at but he's been through so many changes in the last 24 hours. He reorients easily. He has O_2 on at 2L/min via NC, O_2 sats running 90-91, lungs are clear, he gets breathing treatments every 6 hours and PRN, he has COPD. Heart rate irregular in the 70s I think they said. He has a-fib—he is on dig for that. Skin is warm and dry, still got pretty bad skin turgor, abdomen soft with active bowel sounds, no bowel movement since admission. His FBS this morning was 287 and he received coverage with 6 units of Novalog, make sure he eats a good breakfast will you? He has NS at 125 mL/hr into his right hand, it's a #20, site looks good. The pump has beeped a lot-I think it is positional and I told him to keep it up on a pillow. His voiding is good, he has a UTI which is probably what put him into DKA this time. He needs help getting to the bathroom because of the pump and he has a sore foot, we have been assisting him to use the urinal. He is on Fall Precautions. He has an ulcer on his right foot that the wound team has been treating on an outpatient basis, right now we are just doing wet to moist dressing changes BID, I changed the dressing around 2100, there is a surgical consult for it, it looks pretty bad and he might lose part of that foot. He is on IV antibiotics too. He gets one Percocet for the foot pain every 6 hours, last one was at 0120 so he is probably due for another, he rates his pain at a 10 before his meds and a 6-7 afterwards. He might need something besides the Percocet. He had a pretty good night except for the pump, any questions?

4. Organize the patient data from the corrected report into a standardized format using the PACE format. Not all parts will be readily evident in the given scenario but organize the information that you have.

PACE	Corrected Patient Data
P (Patient/Problem)	
A (Assessment/Actions)	
C (Continuing/Changes)	
E (Evaluation)	

■ Melanie goes in and completes a shift assessment on Mr. Devon. She will need to document this information into the electronic health record (EHR).

5. The co-assigned RN states to the student, "I sure miss the paper chart. They were so easy to work with." In comparing the advantages and disadvantages of the two types of charts (paper and electronic) discuss the reasons that a nurse might prefer a paper chart system.

_____

_____

_____

_____

_____

_____

_____

_____

6. The software program used in this facility is a combination of source-oriented and problem-oriented record styles. Describe what each of these formats presents in the health record.

_____

_____

_____

_____

_____

_____

_____

_____

_____

_____

_____

_____

_____

7. Using the following data, document a CBE note and a focus note (DAR) using correct documentation terms and abbreviations. Use the forms provided.

Restless, oriented to person, place, and time. Skin pale, cool, and moist. States, "I don't feel so good and my foot is really hurting me. I didn't feel like much breakfast—it's hard to eat when all you can think about is a painful foot." V/S 149/88 – 98 – 26 – 99.1 O2 sat 94% on 2l/min via NC. Lungs clear bilaterally. Refused scheduled breathing treatment at this time stating to respiratory technician "I just don't feel like it right now." Apical pulse irregularly irregular. Peripheral pulses intact with diminished pedal pulse to right foot. Abdomen soft, round with active bowel sounds. IV NS @ 125 mL/hr via pump to right *hand, site without redness, edema, or tenderness. IV started yesterday. Dressing to right foot dry and intact. Pt states pain is a 10 on a scale of 1–10 and describes it as intense, stabbing pain. States, "I need some pain medication. I should have asked for it earlier though it doesn't seem to help much."*

CBE Entry:

Expected Parameters	WNL*	Notes
Neuromuscular Alert; follows commands; oriented to person, place, and time; opens eyes spontaneously; able to move all extremities with full ROM, handgrips strong and equal; coordinated movements, steady balance and gait; no abnormal sensations or reflexes; face symmetrical; speech clear and coherent; No pain.		
Respirations Respirations regular and unlabored. Symmetrical chest movement. Breath sounds clear bilaterally. Coughs on request, no secretions and on room air. No pain.		
Cardiovascular Heart rhythm regular, heart sounds normal (S_1, S_2), no edema; capillary refill less than 3 seconds. Color normal. No calf tenderness. Radial and pedal pulses palpable 2+ and equal bilaterally. No neck vein distention. No pain.		
Gastrointestinal Abdomen soft, no distention, non-tender. Bowel sounds present in all four quadrants. Formed BM in last 3 days without chemical or mechanical stimulation. No pain.		
Integumentary Warm, dry, intact, elastic turgor. No redness or open areas. No pain.		
IV Therapy/Venous Access IV site without redness, edema, or leakage. Site and tubing within date. Type and rate of fluids documented.		

*Within Normal Limits

DAR Entry:

Date/Time	Focus	Notes
11/29/13 0830	Pain	
0940		

8. The ordered pain medication/schedule is not adequate to treat Mr. Devon's pain. Using the SBAR format, write down how you would discuss this situation with the primary care provider.

S (Situation)	
B (Background)	
A (Assessment)	
R (Recommendations)	

9. You receive the following updated orders via fax from the primary care provider:
- Discontinue Percocet one tab orally every 6 hours prn for pain
- Tylenol #3 one to two tabs orally every 4 hours prn for moderate pain rated at less than a 7 on the pain scale
- Dilaudid 2 mg IV every 4 hours prn for severe pain rated at equal to or greater than 7 on the pain scale

Which order should you question and why?

Vital Signs

After 6 weeks in the nursing arts lab learning basic skills of nursing assessment, Malinda Upchurch is assigned to a medical-surgical nursing unit. Her first day there is to help her acclimate to the unit. She is asked to take the vital signs on the six patients, ranging in age from 51 to 89, assigned to her co-assigned RN.

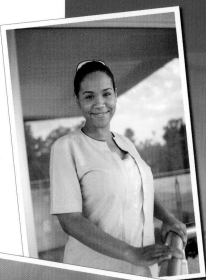

1. What are the expected values of temperature, pulse rate, respirations, and blood pressure for these patients?

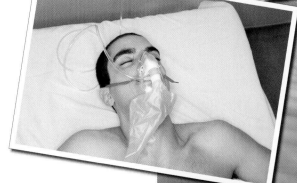

	Oral Temperature Average (Range) °C (°F)	Pulse Average (Range) beats/min	Respirations (Range) breaths/min	Blood Pressure (Average) mm Hg
Adult				
Adult >70 years				

2. What information about the facility equipment does Malinda need before starting her rounds in regard to facility equipment?

_____

_____

_____

_____

_____

3. Discuss the key aspects of infection control when assessing vital signs among a group of patients.

_____

_____

_____

_____

_____

Consider each of the following situations as Malinda completes her rounds on these patients.

- Mrs. Rojas, 84 y.o., does not understand English, with new onset hypertension
- Mr. Oxendine, 51 y.o., on oxygen therapy with a partial rebreather mask for hypoxia breathing rapidly through his mouth
- Mr. Hines, 77 y.o., with congestive heart failure, requiring multiple cardiac medications
- Mrs. Tescarelli, 72 y.o., being evaluated for episodes of syncope
- Mr. Leuong, 89 y.o., confused, with fever from an acute urinary tract infection

4. Discuss each of the following aspects Malinda needs to consider when preparing to measure the vital signs for each of these patients:
   a. Identify factors that may affect each of the measured parameters and the etiology of the change.

Parameter	Factor	Etiology
Temperature		
Pulse		
Respirations		
Blood Pressure		

b. For each patient, which values should Malinda anticipate might be outside the normal parameters? Identify the contributing factors for these variations.

_____

_____

_____

Patient	Temperature	Pulse	Respirations	Blood Pressure
Mrs. Rojas				
Mr. Oxendine				
Mr. Hines				
Mrs. Tescarelli				
Mr. Leuong				

c. Which factor can affect all aspects of vital signs? What does this mean in the provision of nursing care?

_____

_____

_____

_____

d. The facility uses electronic thermometers to assess temperature. Which site, oral, rectal, or axillary, would be best for assessing each patient's temperature? Give a rationale for each choice.

_____

_____

_____

_____

_____

_____

_____

_____

e. If unknown, how would Malinda determine the baseline for inflating the cuff in order to accurately measure the blood pressure?

_____

_____

_____

_____

_____

_____

_____

5. Mr. Leuong's temperature reads at 101.2°F. He is restless and complains of chills. His skin is hot and dry. Four hours ago his temperature was 97.4°F.

a. What is the appropriate nursing diagnosis for this situation?

_____

b. Identify an NOC standardized outcome and individualize it to this patient.

_____

_____

_____

_____

c. Identify two NIC standardized interventions and the specific activities that are appropriate for this patient.

_____

_____

_____

_____

_____

_____

_____

d. The unlicensed person assisting with care tells Malinda, "They put a cooling blanket on him yesterday and we had him shivering that fever out in no time." Discuss this information in view of desired outcomes and evaluation of pyrexia.

_____

_____

_____

6. Mr. Oxendine has a respiratory rate of 28 breaths/min. He states that he feels better after having the "extra oxygen put on" with the mask. He knows that he is being monitored for his breathing. How can Malinda unobtrusively assess his respiratory pattern?

_____

_____

_____

7. To facilitate ease of breathing, what intervention can Malinda easily implement that addresses a factor that influences respirations?

_____

_____

_____

8. As Malinda is going into Mr. Hines's room the co-assigned nurse tells her "Get a full set of pulse characteristics for me will you? I need the apical pulse as well as the peripheral pulses before I give him all his medications and it will be good practice for you. Thanks!"
a. What equipment does she need to complete these tasks?

_____

b. What characteristics should be assessed in the pulses?

_____

_____

_____

_____

_____

_____

_____

_____

c. Is the assessment of the apical-radial pulse indicated in this situation? Why or why not?

_____

_____

_____

_____

_____

d. What is the correct location to auscultate the apical pulse?

_____

_____

e. For patients with congestive heart failure, the heart enlarges due to increased cardiac workload. Picturing the heart as it sits in the chest, would this enlargement change how Malinda would auscultate the apical pulse rate? Why or why not?

_____

_____

_____

_____

_____

_____

9. Upon entering Mrs. Tescarelli's room, Malinda finds her standing at the bedside with the intent of ambulating to the bathroom. Mrs. Tescarelli says, "I sure feel woozy-headed when I get up but I need to go to the bathroom. I know I should ask for help, but you girls are just so busy."

a. Knowing the patient's admission diagnosis, should Malinda immediately take the patient's blood pressure while Mrs. Tescarelli is standing at the bedside? Why or why not?

_____

_____

_____

b. To determine the safety in ambulation for Mrs. Tescarelli, what important assessment should be made prior to ambulation? How should Malinda instruct an unlicensed assistant to complete this task?

_____

_____

_____

c. In monitoring the skill competency of the UAP as he completes the blood pressure measurement using a sphygmomanometer, which of the following steps indicates a need for remediation of this skill? Indicate the correct procedure of that step.
  • Patient positioned on edge of bed with legs dangling freely

  _____

  • Measurement arm placed at heart level
  • Snugly wrapped around the upper arm but avoid discomfort
  • Uses the 200 mm mark as standard for inflation pressure

  _____

  _____

  • Carefully places the diaphragm of the stethoscope under the edge of the cuff.

  _____

  _____

  • Releases cuff pressure slowly at 2–3 mm Hg per second
d. How may the errors skew the blood pressure readings for this patient?

  _____
  _____
  _____
  _____
  _____
  _____

Communication and Therapeutic Relationships

Working in an acute care/rehabilitation center you are assigned as primary nurse to Gabe Huston, an 18-year-old admitted for rehabilitation after sustaining a T-6 spinal cord injury that resulted in paralysis from his waist down. He was also blinded in one eye. He is one of four patients roomed together to enhance socialization and support. Gabe has good family support from his mother and his older brother and he is expected to return to his home and his normal activities with some accommodations after discharge.

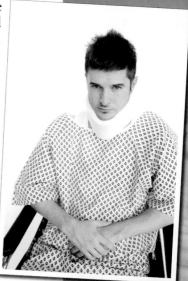

The facility transfer report states that he is still dealing with the loss and is often withdrawn or angry regarding the circumstances. The first interaction often sets the stage for future outcomes of all interactions with the patient.

The key to the therapeutic use of self is your professional communication skills. Effective communication, the exchange of information as well as feelings, is a tool that facilitates the attainment of patient goals in any healthcare setting.

1. Prior to your first interaction during the admission process, consider the many factors that can interfere with effective communication. Discuss how each of the following factors might influence communication with this patient in this setting:
   • Environment
   • Developmental stage
   • Gender
   • Personal space
   • Sociocultural factors
   • Roles and relationships

Factor	Influence on Communication
Environment	
Developmental stage	
Gender	
Personal space	
Sociocultural factors	
Roles and relationships	

2. Upon Gabe's admission to the unit, you need to orient Gabe, as well as his mother and brother, to the routines and expectations of the rehabilitation experience. How can you set the tone of this initial interaction using your understanding of the factors that affect delivery of the message? Discuss the following verbal and non-verbal aspects of communication:
   • Verbal: vocabulary, word meanings, pacing, clarity/brevity, timing, and relevance
   • Non-verbal: posture, gestures, and touch

_____

_____

_____

_____

_____

_____

_____

_____

_____

Gabe's mother and brother have many questions regarding the process and outcomes intended for him. You explain to both Gabe and his family that with a T6-level injury, the expected outcomes include living independently without assistive devices in feeding, bathing, grooming, oral and facial hygiene, dressing, bladder management, and bowel management. He will need a manual wheelchair for mobility but will be able to transfer to/from the chair independently. Gabe remains silent through the orientation process, allowing his family to speak for him.

3. You direct your communication to Gabe and ask him, "What are your thoughts, here at the beginning, about your rehabilitation?" He replies, "It doesn't matter to me. I am never going to walk again so why bother with any of this? I will have to live with my mother the rest of my life and depend on her to take me everywhere and that just #$!!#!" Integrating the key characteristics of empathy, respect, and honesty in therapeutic communication, how would you respond to Gabe? (The response may be several sentences long.)

As Gabe's primary nurse, you begin to work with him every day in supporting his learning through the various therapies that will ensure his optimal independence upon discharge from the facility. His biggest hurdle is acceptance of his need for, and understanding of how to best use, a wheelchair to facilitate his mobility and independence. Prior to his accident Gabe was a cross-country runner in his first year at the university. He states one day while you are preparing his medications, "I don't know why you guys bother with all this. I am never going to be what I used to be." Although he has been compliant with his therapy, this is the first time he has expressed his feelings regarding his outcomes.

4. Using the interventions that enhance therapeutic communication, which techniques would be appropriate for you to use at this time to respond to this statement? Write down a response reflecting the use of the techniques you identified.

_____

_____

_____

_____

_____

_____

_____

_____

_____

It is often easy to put up barriers to communication when interactions are based on social parameters rather than grounded in a framework of a professional therapeutic relationship.

5. For each of the following responses to Gabe's statement, identify the communication barrier and reflect on why a response like that is often used in discussing a patient's concerns.

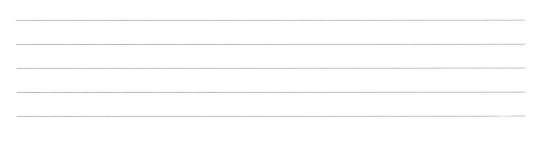

_____

_____

_____

_____

_____

Nurse Response	Communication Barrier	Reflection on Response
"Now, you know you are not a bother at all; it's my job."		
"You are young and will bounce back from this just fine—all you kids do."		
"If I were you I'd take my love of cross-country running and think about doing that with my wheelchair."		
"You should not feel that way. You have so much going for you."		
"Don't worry; you will be even better in a different way when you are done here."		
"Why don't you think you can do things again like you used to? That's the whole purpose of being here."		

6. After a difficult day in therapy, you mention to Gabe the possibility of obtaining a driving evaluation to facilitate his learning to drive a car again with adaptive equipment. He is taken with the idea and asks, "Can you do that—like, now?!" You know that the therapist, Ms. Greene, who manages this case often resents it when other disciplines present information felt to be within her scope of practice. Formulate how you will communicate with this therapist using the SBAR model.

S (Situation)	
B (Background)	
A (Assessment)	
R (Recommendations)	

Health Assessment

Douglas (Dougie) Moore is a 58-year-old patient admitted to your medical unit from a group home for developmentally challenged adults. He is being admitted with bacterial pneumonia. He has Down syndrome and has the developmental level of an 8-year-old. He is in moderate respiratory distress, compounded by anxiety related to admission to an unfamiliar environment. His assigned residence aide has accompanied him to provide reassurance for Dougie per facility policy.

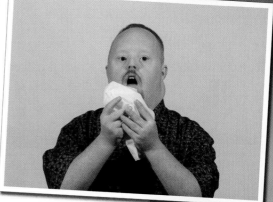

1. Taking Dougie's developmental stage (school age) into consideration, how will this change your approach as you prepare yourself, the environment, and the patient for the examination?

_____

_____

_____

_____

_____

_____

_____

_____

_____

_____

_____

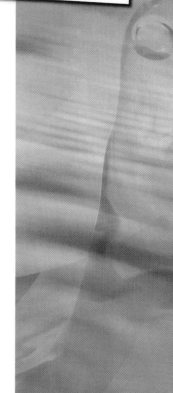

_____

_____

_____

_____

_____

_____

_____

_____

_____

_____

_____

2. How would you explain each of the five techniques of physical examination to Dougie during the examination to allay some of his anxiety?

Technique	Explanation
Inspection	
Palpation	
Percussion	
Auscultation	
Olfaction	

3. In light of Dougie's status, which aspects of the full physical assessment would you defer at this time? Why?

_____

_____

_____

_____

_____

System	Pertinent Assessment Data	Deferred at this time
General physical survey		
Integumentary		
Head		
Neck		
Breasts and axillae		
Chest and lungs		
Cardiovascular		
Abdomen		
Musculoskeletal		
Neurological		
Genitourinary		

4. For each of the following parts of the physical examination, describe the equipment you will need and the procedure/critical points of the assessment.
- Skin color, temperature and turgor, edema
- Pupillary reaction and cardinal fields of gaze
- Mucous membranes
- Breath sounds
- Heart sounds
- Abdomen characteristics
- Bowel sounds
- Capillary refill
- Peripheral pulses

Assessment	Special Equipment	Critical Points
Skin color, Temperature and turgor Edema		
Pupillary reaction Cardinal fields of gaze		
Mucous membranes		
Breath sounds		
Heart sounds		
Abdomen characteristics		

Assessment	Special Equipment	Critical Points
Bowel sounds		
Capillary refill		
Peripheral pulses		

5. The following data are found on the physical examination. Correctly document the findings using correct terminology and professional language.

Dougie knows he is in the hospital because he can't catch his breath and he tells you "my chest hurts when I breathe and I don't feel so good", he is constantly rubbing at his chest, blue-gray color to lips and facial features, hot feel to skin, pinched skin on back of hand stays in place, swelling in feet, pressure makes an indent of about 1/8 inch which fills in rapidly when pressure removed, pale color to nail beds, when pinched pink color comes back quickly, small mouth with tongue sticking out, mucous membranes dry looking, lungs with snoring, continuous low pitched sounds when breathing in and out, spitting out sticky green yellow sputum, breathing at 28 breaths per minute, working at breathing, apical pulse heard in correct anatomical position with no extra noises, pulses in neck, wrists, legs and feet easily felt, belly normal shape without pain, rumbling noted at regular intervals in all areas of abdomen

_____

_____

_____

_____

_____

_____

_____

_____

Promoting Asepsis and Preventing Infection

You and a classmate are assigned to assist in meeting the self-care/hygiene needs for the following group of post-operative hip surgery patients on the orthopedic surgery/ rehabilitation unit.

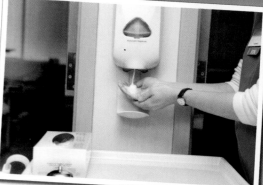

- Mr. Joseph Hernandez, 74 years old, right hip replacement, history of lung disease, suspected of having influenza, on droplet isolation
- Ms. Pamela Guy, 91 years old, left hip replacement, has dementia, must be fed all meals
- Mrs. Edna Watson, 84 years old, left hip fracture repair, positive for MRSA in her urine, on contact precautions
- Mrs. Alicia Flowers, 89 years old, right hip replacement, currently receiving chemotherapy for skin cancer, on protective isolation
- Mr. Frank Centralli, 67 years old, left hip replacement for degenerative joint disease, history of smoking 3 ppd × 45 years
- Ms. Ruth McNally, 87 years old, right hip fracture repair secondary to a fall at home, history of diabetes and hypertension

For all the patients, attention to promoting asepsis and preventing infection is a mainstay of safe patient care. For the assigned patients, consider each of the following key aspects during your provision of basic care and comfort measures:

1. Describe each link in the chain of infection

Links	Description
Infectious agent	
Reservoir	
Portal of exit	
Mode of transmission	
Portal of entry	
Susceptible host	

2. Discuss the commonalties of the assigned patients' risk for development of an infection based on your understanding of the chain of infection.

_____

_____

_____

_____

_____

_____

_____

_____

_____

_____

_____

_____

3. What key indicators can be assessed that would indicate the use of the body's secondary defenses in response to pathogen invasion?

_____

_____

_____

4. Differentiate the two types of specific immunity that make up a patient's tertiary defenses by the following characteristics:
a. Type of lymphocyte
b. Site of action
c. Method of protection

	Humoral Immunity	Cell-Mediated Immunity
Type of Lymphocyte		
Site of Action		
Method of Protection		

5. Based on an understanding of the lifestyle factors which support the patients' own host defenses against infection, what interventions can you identify that are within your scope of practice as a nursing student?

Lifestyle Factor	Interventions
Nutrition	
Hygiene	

Lifestyle Factor	Interventions
Rest & Exercise	
Stress Reduction	

6. Which factors in the physiology of each of the assigned patients increase the risk for infection during this hospitalization? List the eight factors in the left column of the table.

Factor	Hernandez	Guy	Watson	Flowers	Centralli	McNally

7. Which diagnostic testing results should be monitored for ongoing assessment of Mrs. Watson's infection and response to treatment?

8. In implementing hygiene modalities, how do the mandates of medical asepsis fit into the care measures for these patients?

Standard Precautions

- Immediately wash your hands with soap and water after contact with blood, body fluids (except sweat), excretions and secretions, mucous membranes, any break in the skin, or contaminated objects REGARDLESS of whether you have been wearing gloves.
- Wear clean gloves whenever there is potential for contact with blood, body fluids, secretions, excretions, non-intact skin, or contaminated materials.
- Remove gloves immediately after use. Avoid touching clean items, environmental surfaces, or another patient.
- Change gloves between tasks or procedures on the same patient if you have made contact with material that may contain a high concentration of microorganisms.
- Wash your hands with soap and water after removing gloves, between patient contacts, and between procedures on the same patient to prevent cross-contamination of different body sites.
- Wear a mask and eye protection or a face shield to protect mucous membranes of the eyes, nose, and mouth during patient care activities that are likely to generate splashes or sprays of blood, body fluids, secretions, and excretions.
- Wear a clean, non-sterile gown to protect skin and prevent soiling of clothing whenever there is a risk of spray or splash onto clothing. Promptly remove the gown once it is soiled. Avoid contaminating clothing when removing the gown. Wash hands after removing the gown.
- Clean reusable equipment that is soiled with blood or body fluids according to agency policy.
- Do not reuse equipment for the care of another patient until it has been cleaned and reprocessed appropriately.
- Dispose of single-use equipment that is soiled with blood or body fluids in appropriate biohazard containers.
- Carefully handle contaminated linens to prevent skin and mucous membrane exposures, contamination of clothing, and transfer of microorganism to other patients or the environment.

9. What will be different when providing care for Mrs. Watson, Mr. Hernandez, and Mrs. Flowers?

_____

_____

_____

_____

_____

_____

_____

_____

_____

_____

_____

_____

10. How can the key procedures of surgical asepsis impact care for patients on this surgical unit?

11. Mrs. Flowers states, "I just feel so alone in my room." Discuss the interventions that address this verbalized need.

_____

_____

_____

12. Based on your understanding of the knowledge and practice base for the promotion of asepsis and prevention of infection, use the Critical-Thinking Model (CTM) to approach your patient care assignment so that you and your classmates are well prepared and able to function safely in meeting your patient's self-care/hygiene needs.

_____

_____

_____

_____

_____

_____

_____

_____

_____

_____

_____

_____

_____

_____

_____

_____

_____

_____

13. How does the infection control nurse contribute to the institutional goal of promoting asepsis and preventing infection in regard to both the institution and its healthcare workers?

_____

_____

_____

_____

_____

_____

_____

14. How can the nurse facilitate surveillance of infection in the community setting?

_____

_____

_____

_____

_____

_____

_____

_____

_____

_____

Safety: Falls

■ Thad Lutz is a 54 y.o. admitted for a deep vein thrombosis (DVT) of the left leg. Five days ago, he had surgery for a left ruptured Achilles tendon sustained during a local 10K race. He has never been hospitalized prior to his outpatient surgery. Post-operative instructions include no weight-bearing on the left leg for 4 weeks. He has crutches, but admits instead to "hopping around at home holding onto things" on his right leg. He has an IV line via infusion pump for heparin therapy for anticoagulation. He still requires oral pain medication for post-operative pain compounded by the pain of the DVT. He is on complete bedrest with allowed use of a bedside commode (BSC).

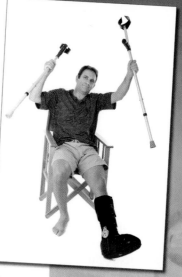

1. As part of the routine admission assessment, a Morse Fall Scale is completed. Explain the variables that pertain to Mr. Lutz for this admission.

_____

_____

_____

_____

_____

_____

_____

_____

_____

_____

_____

2. After reviewing the Medicare "never events," which ones could present a risk to Mr. Lutz during this hospitalization?

_____

3. The nurse identifies a potential diagnosis of Risk for falls[†] related to imbalanced gait with an outcome of no episodes of falls during hospitalization. The nurse discusses the diagnosis with Mr. Lutz, but he does not view falling as a hazard. He states, "I am young and in great shape and getting around on one leg works just fine for me." How would you approach this perspective so that a collaborative plan of care can be implemented with this patient?

_____
_____
_____
_____
_____
_____
_____
_____
_____
_____

Despite agreement on measures to ensure his safety, Mr. Lutz continues to "ambulate" to the bathroom without assistance instead of using the BSC. He uses the infusion pump and its rolling stand for balance and tells the nursing assistant that he does not want to bother anyone when he can figure it all out on his own. The nursing assistant tells the nurse, "That man needs to be tied down before he hurts himself."

4. With the knowledge that Mr. Lutz still needs pain medication every 4 to 6 hours, would any kind of restraint be appropriate in this situation? Explain your rationale.

_____
_____
_____
_____
_____
_____
_____
_____

[†]© 2012 NANDA International

5. Recognizing that pain medications can impair cognition, discuss the interventions that you can put in place to avoid the need for restraints for this patient.

6. It is decided to implement the use of a bed exit alarm for Mr. Lutz. How will this device help decrease the incidence of falls for this patient?

_____
_____
_____
_____

7. The nursing assistant tells you, "I don't know how to use one of those." How would you demonstrate and instruct the assistant on how to implement a bed exit alarm?

_____
_____
_____
_____
_____
_____
_____
_____

8. What important teaching points should be communicated to Mr. Lutz?

_____
_____

Mr. Lutz has recovered from his DVT, is regulated on his warfarin sodium (Coumadin) therapy, an oral anticoagulant medication, and is ready for discharge. Discharge instructions are completed with him and his wife regarding medications, pain control, and ambulation parameters. His wife states, "I sure hope he behaves. I bet he didn't tell you he fell several times at the house trying to hop around on his good foot."

9. Discuss six key points with Mr. and Mrs. Lutz concerning the prevention of falls in the home.

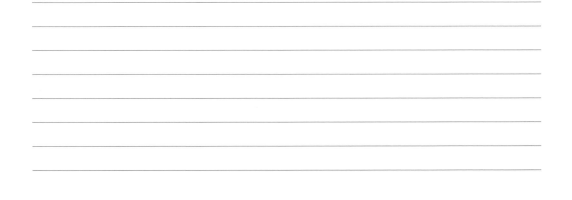

10. In addition, Mrs. Lutz explains that her elderly father-in-law lives with them. She worries about his ability to get around safely and asks you, "How can I know if Dad is at risk for falls? He's as stubborn as his son!" Explain the "Get Up and Go Test" to Mrs. Lutz.

_____

_____

_____

_____

_____

Self-Care Ability: Hygiene

Ms. Juanita Morganson and Ms. Hannah Lithgrow are nursing students co-assigned to care for a resident during their long-term care rotation. They will be working with this resident for 5 weeks. Based on the assessment of functional abilities as well as data gathered through the assessment guidelines for hygiene, they are to implement a plan of care to meet the self-care needs of the resident.

■ Addie Johnson is a 52-year-old morbidly obese female with diabetes mellitus. She has had a stroke and has right-sided paralysis (hemiplegia). She tends to slow, cautious behavior and needs frequent instruction and feedback to complete tasks. She has retinopathy (affects her eyesight) and peripheral neuropathy (affects sensation in legs) from her diabetes mellitus. Her Katz Index of Independence in Activities of Daily Living indicates that she is very dependent in the areas of bathing, dressing, transferring, and toileting.

1. Discuss how this resident's health status has affected her self-care ability.

_____

_____

_____

_____

2. During assessment of self-care, the students consult with the resident to assess her willingness and ability to perform ADLs. Why is this step vital to the plan of care and how will it affect the completion of hygiene care for this resident?

_____

_____

_____

_____

The initial interview with Ms. Johnson elicits the following information from the resident:

- "I can't do anything for myself without a lot of help since my right side doesn't work."
- "My sugars have really made me sick over the years; it has affected my eyes and my feet."
- "I want to help take care of myself but I am just too slow at it and I will admit my size makes it hard."
- "I've always taken my bath before I went to bed but here I am on the Thursday morning bath list, with 'spot washes' in between. They use the shower chair and have me scrubbed up in no time. It's just easier for the girls here."

3. For each of the responses given by Ms. Johnson, write an open-ended question to elicit more detail to her responses. Why is this important to the development of an individualized plan of care for this resident?

Patient Response	Examples of Open-Ended Questions
"I can't do anything for myself without a lot of help since my right side doesn't work."	
"My sugars have really made me sick over the years; it has affected my eyes and my feet."	
"I want to help take care of myself but I am just too slow at it and sometimes I forget what I am doing."	
"I've always taken my bath before I went to bed but here I am on the Thursday morning bath list, with 'spot washes' in between. They use the shower chair and have me scrubbed up in no time. It's just easier for the girls here."	

_____

_____

_____

_____

_____

4. The students identify a nursing diagnosis of Bathing/Hygiene Self-Care Deficit[†] for Ms. Johnson. Based on the initial interview data as well as potential responses to the follow-up questions write a three-part nursing diagnostic statement to reflect this individual need of this resident.

_____

_____

Using the Assessment Guidelines, hygiene, the following data are documented regarding Ms. Johnson's physical status as it relates to hygiene needs:

Topic	Assessment Data
Environment	Room warm, "stuffy," stale odors
Skin	Ashen gray color, skin moist, red rash that "burns and itches" present under both breasts, skin folds on abdomen, in both axilla, crevices of groin, musty odor to areas, shiny, thin skin to lower extremities, receiving treatment for fungal infections of the skin
Feet	Dry, reddened area to right heel, moist reddened skin between toes
Nails	Hard, thick toenails
Oral Cavity	Lips smooth and pink, oral mucosa and gums pink, moist, wears upper and lower dentures, teeth aligned well, pairs in chewing position, redness noted on left lower gum under dentures, "sore"
Hair	Dry, coarse hair at present contained in braids, scalp dry, no lesions
Eyes	Wears glasses to read, history of diabetic retinopathy, no redness or drainage

5. Based on Ms. Johnson's capabilities, which type of bath would best fit this situation and why?

_____

_____

_____

_____

_____

6. Ms. Johnson tells you during the bath, "In the hospital they had prepackaged bath kits. I wish they had them here. I could do parts myself using them." These products are not available in this facility. How could you provide a similar experience for this resident?

7. During the partial baths done in her room, how would you ensure privacy, safety, and comfort for this resident? Think: What would you desire if you were in this same situation?

8. In addition to the medication ordered by the primary care provider to address Ms. Johnson's fungal infections of the skin, what other interventions can be done to decrease the skin problems associated with being morbidly obese that are individualized to this resident?

_____

_____

_____

_____

_____

_____

_____

_____

_____

_____

_____

_____

9. What kind of positioning, skin care, and procedural steps would you need to implement to provide adequate/individualized perineal care for Ms. Johnson?

_____

_____

_____

_____

_____

_____

_____

_____

_____

10. The charge nurse asks the students to complete the Brief Oral Health Status Examination (BOHSE). Based on the information that has been obtained through the hygiene assessment, what would you expect the results of this examination to be? What further interventions are needed at this time based on the results?

_____

_____

_____

_____

_____

_____

Medication Administration

You have been assigned to be the medication nurse in a long-term care facility to a group of 20 residents, of which 7 are there for short-term rehabilitation after total hip replacement. It is the first time you have worked with this group and therefore are unfamiliar with their medication routines and preferences.

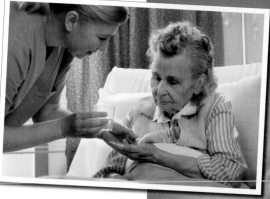

1. The 1900–0730 shift nurse has completed his report and asks you if there are any questions. What information regarding the residents themselves would be beneficial for you to know in order to organize the administration of medications for the shift?

_____

_____

_____

_____

_____

_____

_____

_____

_____

_____

2. The distribution system for this facility is a combination of stock supply and unit dose. Why would these two systems be most appropriate for a long-term care facility?

_____

_____

_____

_____

_____

_____

_____

The Medication Administration Record (MAR) for one of your assigned residents, Mrs. Lowery, is provided for you to use for your shift 0700–1930.

3. For medications you are unfamiliar with, what resources could you use to learn about these medications prior to administration? Which one is the best source of nursing implications?

_____

_____

_____

_____

_____

4. The MAR reflects the "standard" administration times used in the facility when transcribing the medication orders. Based on an understanding of pharmacodynamics and medication interactions for the oral medications, which administration times are not appropriate? Explain.

_____

_____

_____

_____

_____

_____

_____

_____

_____

5. Using an SBAR format, how would you approach the primary care provider to address this issue?

S (Situation)	
B (Background)	
A (Assessment)	
R (Recommendations)	

6. For each of the medications listed on the MAR:
   a. What equipment will you need to prepare and administer the medications?
   b. What key physical assessments and/or lab data are needed prior to administering these medications?

Medication	Route	Equipment	Patient/Lab Data
Nitro-Dur patch			
NovoLog			
Lanoxin			
Caltrate			
Coumadin			
Lyrica			

(Continued)

Medication	Route	Equipment	Patient/Lab Data
Actonel			
Timoptic			
Combivent			
Cyanocobalamin			

7. Describe the "Rights of Medication" and the "Three Checks." How do these facilitate a culture of safety in medication administration?

Right	Key Points
Drug	
Patient	
Dose	
Route	
Time	
Documentation	
Reason	
To Know	
To Refuse	

_____

_____

_____

_____

_____

_____

_____

_____

_____

8. Mrs. Lowery tells you, "I am not taking all those nine o'clock pills. I can't swallow them—they get stuck in my throat."

a. What information do you need about the ordered medications to address this problem?

_____

_____

_____

_____

_____

b. What alternatives are available to help with this swallowing issue?

Medication	Usual Dosage Form	Can It Be Crushed?	Alternatives
Caltrate with vitamin D			
Lyrica			

c. How would you administer the medications to Mrs. Lowery?

_____

_____

_____

9. The medication Lyrica is not available in the resident's routine medication drawer. What could be the cause of this problem and how will you obtain the medication when needed?

_____

_____

_____

_____

_____
_____
_____
_____

10. You go to place the Nitro-Dur patch on Mrs. Lowery and note that the patch from yesterday is still applied to her chest. The MAR indicates that it was removed the previous evening as ordered. What should be your first action? How will you address this occurrence?

_____
_____
_____
_____
_____
_____
_____
_____
_____
_____
_____
_____
_____
_____
_____
_____
_____

11. Mrs. Lowery prefers to insert her own eye drops. As you observe her doing so, what key aspects of the administration procedure should she be doing to ensure correct technique?

_____
_____
_____
_____
_____

12. Mrs. Lowery refuses the extender or spacer for her Combivent inhaler, telling you, "It's too much trouble." How would you explain the benefits of its use to her?

_____

_____

_____

_____

_____

13. The cyanocobalamin solution is provided in a vial with a concentration of 1 mg/1 mL.
  a. Calculate the correct volume for the ordered dose.

  b. What type of syringe and needle gauge will you use for administration? Are there others that can also be used for this? Explain.

_____

_____

_____

_____

_____

_____

_____

  c. Where will you administer this injection? Give a rationale for your choice.

_____

_____

_____

_____

_____

d. How can you minimize the discomfort of the injection for Mrs. Lowery?

_____

_____

_____

_____

_____

_____

_____

_____

_____

14. Mrs. Lowery tells you, "I always have an allergic reaction to this drug. I get diarrhea for a few days each month after I get it." What information do you need and how would you address this concern?

_____

_____

_____

_____

_____

_____

_____

_____

_____

_____

_____

_____

_____

_____

_____

_____

_____

RESIDENT: Mrs. Elizabeth Lowery	**DOB:** 03/27/1926		**PAGE 1 of 1**

Medical Hx: early onset dementia, atrial fibrillation COPD, IDDM, glaucoma, hx left hip fx w/ORIF, MI, cardiac pacemaker, MRSA

Precautions: Falls, Aspiration   **ALLERGIES:** Latex, Penicillin, Sulfa drugs

Codes for Injection Sites		Initials	Signature/Title
A: Left deltoid	1: Right deltoid		
B: Left lateral arm	2: Right lateral arm		
C: Left ventral arm	3: Right ventral arm		
D: Left anterior thigh	4: Right anterior thigh		
E: Left lateral thigh	5: Right lateral thigh		
F: Left ventrogluteal	6: Right ventrogluteal		
G: Left upper abdomen	7: Right upper abdomen		
H: Left lower abdomen	8: Right lower abdomen		
I: Left upper back	9: Right upper back		

Medication	Hour	Day Of The Month																														
		1	2	3	4	5	6	7	8	9	10	11	12	13	14	15	16	17	18	19	20	21	22	23	24	25	26	27	28	29	30	31
Nitro-Dur patch 0.2 mg/hr to skin daily	0900																															
Nitro-Dur patch REMOVED at HS	2100																															
Novolog 70/30 24 units Subq daily ac breakfast	0730 / site																															
Novolog 70/30 12 units Subq daily ac dinner	1630 / site																															
Lanoxin 0.25 mg daily at 1700	1700 AP rate																															
Caltrate 500 mg with Vitamin D TID	0900 / 1500 / 2100																															
Coumadin 3 mg daily at 1700	1700																															
Donepezil 5 mg daily HS	2100																															
Combivent 2 puffs QID with MDI	0900 / 1300 / 1700 / 2100																															
Actonel 5 mg daily	0900																															
Timoptic 1 drop to both eyes BID	0900 / 2100																															
Lyrica 50 mg TID	0900 / 1500 / 2100																															
Cyanocobalamin 200 mcg IM monthly	0900 / site	X	X	X	X	X	X	X	X	X	X	X	X	X	X	X	X	X	X	X	X	X	X	X	X	X	X	X	X	X	X	X

Teaching and Learning

Haley is a 7-year-old girl who received a new percutaneous endoscopic gastrostomy (PEG). Due to having eosinophilic esophagitis (EE), she has been unable to maintain an adequate nutritional status for healthy growth and development and it was decided that supplemental enteral feedings would be beneficial. Her primary caregiver is her 72-year-old grandmother, Mary, who has cared for Haley since she was 3 months old. Haley will be receiving bolus feedings as well as two medications through the PEG. As the primary nurse you are responsible 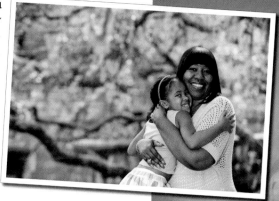 for development and implementation of a teaching plan for this family system.

Mary has expressed to you that "I've never seen anything like this before. I hope I can do this right. They want to send us home soon and I just want to be ready. I don't want to hurt my baby by doing it wrong. When the doctor was telling me everything, it seems hard to do but I want what is best for Haley. It is a relief in a way to finally have a way to help Haley feel better and grow better. She has been sick for so long. I want this to be a 'fun thing' for Haley and I know once it settles in she will feel better too. I don't have a lot of learning, I left school in the 6th grade, but I know we can figure this out. I didn't get a lot of what the doctor was telling me about the whole thing here, she talked so fast and I don't hear real well, but I want to get this, OK? I will need to see it and do it a lot to be good at it. I am used to

Supporting Physiological Functioning

UNIT 4

Stress-Coping-Adaptation

During her first semester of nursing school, Tanisha Egwu made friends with another student, who like herself, was juggling work and family responsibilities along with school. Tanisha did well the first semester while her friend struggled with the academic rigors of the program. This semester, she has found herself assigned to the same clinical group as her friend. To help her friend get a good start to the semester, she agreed to work together in preparing their clinical assignments the night before they were due and, at the insistence of her friend, carpool to the clinical site together. Tanisha is somewhat apprehensive about the effect this may have on her own studies, as her friend tends to disorganization in her schoolwork as well as in other areas of her life. At present Tanisha's husband is overseas with the

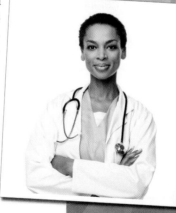

military and her mother-in-law is reluctantly helping with the care of her 4-year-old and 10-month-old children. Her mother-in-law feels that Tanisha should be home to care for the children instead of "selfishly running off to school when my son is serving honorably overseas." Tanisha's husband is supportive of her school studies. Tanisha works one day a week at an assisted living center as a medication technician to help with income issues. Prior to school

219

she was employed full-time as a bookkeeper for a car dealership. Last month she was selected by the facility as employee of the month. It was the staff there that encouraged her and now supports her studies to get her nursing degree.

1. Using the Homes-Rahe Social Readjustment Scale, what are the stressors for Tanisha in the past year and the percentage score representing the chance of a major illness for Tanisha at this time in her life?

_____

_____

_____

_____

_____

_____

_____

_____

_____

_____

_____

_____

_____

_____

2. For the stressors identified by the scale, determine the category of stress they represent in her life. (A stressor may fit in more than one category.)

Category of Stress	Stressors
Distress	
Eustress	
External	
Internal	

Category of Stress	Stressors
Developmental	
Situational	
Physiological	
Psychological	

As the semester progresses, Tanisha is enjoying her nursing studies but growing concerned about her friend in the program. After a long day in clinical her friend tells Tanisha, "What a day in clinical! The instructor was checking me every second of the day! I am pretty good but I can't look good with *you* in the group."

3. Which psychological defense mechanism is being used?

_____

_____

4. How should Tanisha respond to this statement?

_____

_____

_____

_____

_____

The next week Tanisha finds herself apprehensive about attending clinical with her friend. They did their clinical preparation together at the hospital the evening before, although her friend was over an hour late, explaining that her babysitter was running late for the evening. She told Tanisha, "I wish I had live-in help like you do with your mother-in-law." In addition, she told her that she had not been feeling well due to "some kind of GI bug." Tanisha tries to bolster a can-do attitude in her friend regarding the experience the following day, to which her friend responds, "It's just up to the cosmos, I guess, and I'll just have to go along with it. I think they have decided I am not going to do well." This is different from Tanisha's outlook in that she feels that the better the preparation, the more apt she is to do well and she looks forward to clinical.

5. Describe how the personal factors influencing adaptation to the stressors of clinical differ for these two students.

Factor	Tanisha	Friend
Perception		
Overall health status		
Support system		
Hardiness		
Other personal factors		

6. Tanisha's apprehension for her friend continues into the morning of clinical when she arrives a few minutes late to their established carpool routine and states, "I had to stop and go to the bathroom three times on the way here and I've been sick all night." When Tanisha asks, "Do you think you feel OK to take care of patients today?" her friend erupts in anger and then dissolves into tears, stating, "I just don't know why all this is happening; it seems I have been sick since the beginning of the semester. I just don't know if I am going to make it—I just can't handle all this at once." Discuss the behavioral and physiological responses the friend is experiencing in relation to the stress of her nursing program.

_____

_____

_____

_____

_____

_____

_____

7. It is obvious to Tanisha that her friend is in crisis. Using the goals of crisis intervention, how should Tanisha address this situation?

_____

Goals	Example of Response

After resolution of the situation, Tanisha recognizes that she too has a lot of stress in her life related to her many responsibilities and she wants to be able to deal proactively with the stress. She seeks assistance from the student health center/counseling services. The nurse practitioner (NP) identifies a nursing diagnosis with Tanisha of Readiness for Enhanced Coping.[†]

8. Identify an appropriate NOC outcome for Tanisha that reflects her desire to implement measures for stress mitigation through supporting coping abilities. Write two individualized outcomes for Tanisha.

_____

_____

_____

_____

_____

_____

Together, Tanisha and the NP identify an NIC standardized intervention of Coping Enhancement. Most stress-relieving interventions work by one or more of the following means:

• Removing or modifying the stressors
• Supporting coping abilities
• Treating the person's responses to stress

9. Reviewing Tanisha's information, discuss which of the stress-relieving interventions are relevant to this situation.

_____

_____

_____

_____

_____

_____

_____

_____

_____

_____

_____

_____

10. With an understanding of Tanisha's busy lifestyle and etiology of her stressors, discuss the health promotion activities that would be most appropriate for her to implement.

Nutrition

As part of his clinical rotation, Sean Martin is assigned to work with the nutritional support team at the hospital. The team includes a registered nurse, registered dietitian, pharmacist, and medical physician. Patients with actual or potential nutritional issues are referred to this team for management of their nutritional care as well as support for those caring for these patients including the nursing staff and family.

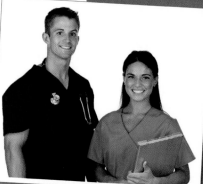

The census list for consultation for the day's rotation includes the following patients:

- Mrs. Sharon Feinstein, an 81-year-old female with dementia and weight loss
- Mr. Adam Belcher, a 37-year-old male with severe hypertension
- Ms. Amelia Stroupe, a 77-year-old female with right-sided weakness and mild dysphagia
- Ms. Michelle Ryan, a 42-year-old female with difficulty breathing secondary to exacerbation of COPD

Ms. Ryan tells you, "I just don't have much of an appetite anymore and I know I need to eat to get better."

1. What measures can you delegate to the nursing assistant to stimulate the patient's appetite at mealtimes?

_____

_____

_____

_____

_____

_____

_____

_____

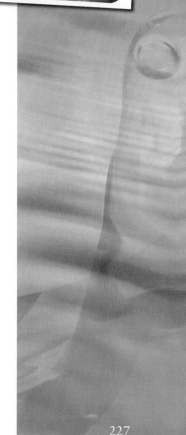

_____
_____
_____
_____
_____
_____
_____
_____
_____
_____

2. How does dyspnea affect the attainment of adequate nutrition? What strategies can be employed to help with this? Consider the aspects discussed in stimulating a patient's appetite as well as information found in caring for patients with oxygenation problems.

_____
_____
_____
_____
_____
_____
_____
_____
_____
_____
_____
_____

The nurse tells Sean that Mrs. Feinstein has the characteristics of malnutrition.

3. What results would support this interpretation? Consider applicable laboratory and body composition data.

_____
_____
_____
_____

_____
_____
_____
_____
_____
_____
_____
_____
_____
_____
_____
_____
_____
_____
_____
_____

4. What physical assessment data should Sean anticipate finding in this situation?

_____
_____
_____
_____
_____
_____
_____
_____
_____
_____

The family wishes to try trial feedings for 6 weeks to enhance her quality of life. Orders are received to place a feeding tube in preparation for enteral feedings.

5. Which type of feeding tube is indicated for this situation? Why?

_____
_____
_____

_____
_____
_____
_____

6. The primary care provider orders a 12 Fr nasogastric tube to be inserted for the feeding trial. What equipment will Sean need to complete this procedure with this patient?

_____
_____
_____
_____
_____
_____
_____
_____
_____
_____
_____

7. What modifications in the procedural steps will Sean need to make, considering Mrs. Feinstein's dementia?

_____
_____
_____
_____
_____
_____
_____
_____
_____
_____
_____
_____

8. Which bedside techniques to check for tube placement are appropriate for this patient situation? Give rationales for your choices. Why did you exclude the techniques that you did?

Mrs. Stroupe has been placed on aspiration precautions.

9. How should Sean implement this during meal times?

10. The nurse identifies the nursing diagnosis of Risk for aspiration.[†] The outcome is aspiration prevention. Write two individualized outcomes that would demonstrate attainment of this goal.

_____

_____

_____

_____

11. Mrs. Stroupe is encouraged to be as independent as possible at meals. Discuss how Sean can best assist with feeding success in this situation.

_____

_____

_____

_____

Mr. Belcher needs dietary instruction in regard to calorie reduction and sodium restriction.

12. He comments to Sean, "I just don't feel like I am that overweight like the doctor says I am. I've always been big boned and played football—I still do some pickup games. I am 6 feet tall and only 265 pounds and in great shape." What is this patient's BMI? How would you explain it to this patient?

_____

_____

_____

_____

_____

_____

_____

13. Describe how you would teach him how to use the MyPlate strategy to manage his nutritional intake.

Recommended resources:

http://www.cnpp.usda.gov/Publications/MyPlate/GettingStartedWithMyPlate.pdf

http://www.choosemyplate.gov/myplate/index.aspx

_____

_____

_____

_____

14. How should Sean respond when he states, "I am thinking about switching to a vegetarian diet because I hear it is a healthier way to eat. How does it change this MyPlate strategy you told me about?"

http://www.choosemyplate.gov/healthy-eating-tips/tips-for-vegetarian.html

http://www.choosemyplate.gov/food-groups/downloads/TenTips/

DGTipsheet8HealthyEatingFor-Vegetarians.pdf

15. In addition he asks, "How do I know how much salt I am really getting?" Discuss how Sean should teach this patient about reading nutrition labels for sources of salt.

_____

_____

_____

_____

_____

_____

_____

_____

Elimination: Urinary

The change of shift report tells you that Ms. Priscilla Barnes, a 47-year-old, admitted with acute asthma, had a restless night. She is still dyspneic at 28 breaths/min and still demonstrating inspiratory and expiratory wheezes, although not as acute as they were at admission. She is maintaining an oxygen saturation of 90% to 92% on oxygen at 4 L/min via nasal cannula. She is receiving breathing treatments every six hours and but needed a prn treatment around 0300. She is receiving IV fluids of NS at 150 mL/hr and an aminophylline drip at 35 mL/hr.

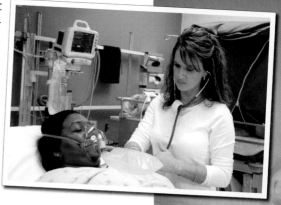

As you enter the room to do your shift assessment, Ms. Barnes tells you, "I don't know what is going on with me. I have to go to the bathroom all the time and I just can't make it there. I am so embarrassed—I just wet myself and the bed. I can't catch my breath when I get up plus I can't get there fast enough with all this stuff attached to me."

1. What should be your initial response to Ms. Barnes?

_____

_____

_____

_____

_____

_____

2. You identify a nursing diagnosis of Urinary incontinence, functional[†] for this patient. Based on the patient information, identify the defining characteristics that validate this diagnosis.

_____

_____

_____

_____

_____

_____

_____

3. She asks you, "Why do I have to go to the bathroom so much?" How would you respond?

_____

_____

_____

_____

_____

_____

4. What would you expect the characteristics and specific gravity of her urine to be, considering her situation?

_____

_____

_____

_____

_____

5. What "at risk" nursing diagnoses might need to be addressed for this patient care situation related to the problem of functional urinary incontinence?

_____

_____

_____

_____

_____

_____

_____

_____

_____

_____

_____

_____

_____

_____

A toileting schedule is created to ensure that Ms. Barnes has adequate opportunity to void, therefore preventing episodes of incontinence.

6. Due to Ms. Barnes's dyspnea, it is decided to have her use a bedpan rather than ambulating to the bathroom. How can you make this modality comfortable for Ms. Barnes? Consider both the physiological and psychosocial aspects of voiding.

_____

_____

_____

_____

_____

_____

_____

_____

_____

_____

_____

_____

Despite the interventions for her asthma, Ms. Barnes's respiratory status deteriorates and she is unable to use the bedpan without compromising her oxygenation status. You receive an order to insert an indwelling catheter to bedside drainage to monitor and manage her urinary output.

7. What type of catheter will you choose to use for this intervention? Why?

_____

_____

_____

8. How will you prepare Ms. Barnes both physically and psychologically for this procedure?

_____

_____

_____

_____

_____

_____

_____

9. Ms. Barnes states, "I have to sit straight up or I can't catch my breath—please don't lay me down flat." How will this affect the catheterization procedure for this patient?

_____

_____

_____

_____

_____

_____

_____

_____

_____

_____

10. In reviewing the steps of catheterization, discuss why organization is key to implementation of this procedure for this patient.

_____

_____

_____

_____

_____

_____

_____

11. You write a nursing order for catheter care q8h for Ms. Barnes. What aspects of this order can be delegated to the nursing assistant?

Goals of Catheter Care	Aspects That Can Be Delegated to the UAP

12. During the shift you offer to assist the assigned aide, to help Ms. Barnes to move up in the bed. The aide places Ms. Barnes flat in the bed and carefully lays the drainage bag next to her thigh so it does not get pulled on during the repositioning, as this will cause discomfort. She instructs the patient to pull her knees up to help push with her feet and on the count of 3, you and the aide, using the drawsheet, pull Ms. Barnes up in the bed. The patient is placed back in high Fowler's position and you ensure that the call light is within reach. The patient is appreciative of this reposi- tioning. Which aspects of this task, if any, indicate that review of this basic patient care task needs to be done with the nursing assistant? Explain.

13. Ms. Barnes's respiratory status improves and you receive an order to remove the catheter. What equipment will you need to implement this order? With the under- standing of the Centers for Disease Control and Prevention (CDC) guidelines on prevention of catheter-associated urinary tract infections (CAUTI), are sterile gloves indicated for this procedure? Give the rationale for your decision.

14. After 8 hours Ms. Barnes is still unable to void post-catheter removal. She does not complain of discomfort and there is no abdominal distention. What measures can you implement to facilitate voiding?

15. During the evening medication rounds, Ms. Barnes says to you, "I sure hope I don't get an infection like I did with that catheter after my second baby was born. I was so miserable when I got home from the hospital. I know that was a long time ago but I sure do remember how miserable I was and it seems I have been prone to them ever since." Discuss the teaching you need to implement with her in the prevention of and/or surveillance for urinary tract infections.

Bowel Elimination: Constipation

You are the nurse in the student health center on the university campus. Sasha Wilkins, a freshman student, comes into the center 2 weeks into her first semester complaining of abdominal pain and states "I don't feel good—there is something wrong with my stomach."

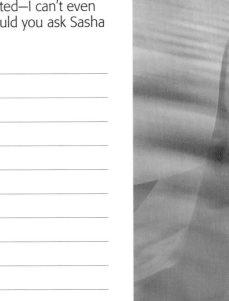

1. Construct a broad opening statement that would encourage more information regarding her complaint.

_____

_____

2. Sasha tells the nurse, "My stomach is so bloated—I can't even button my jeans." What further questions should you ask Sasha to focus on bowel functioning?

_____

_____

_____

_____

_____

_____

_____

_____

_____

3. You need to do a focused physical assessment for bowel elimination. Explain to Sasha how you will proceed. Defer the palpation of the anus and rectum at this time.

_____

_____

_____

_____

_____

_____

_____

_____

_____

_____

The physical assessment reveals that Sasha has a hard, distended abdomen with hypoactive bowel sounds. Percussion and palpation reveal a hard, distended descending colon in the left lower quadrant. She is extremely embarrassed and tells you, "I haven't gone to the bathroom in 9 days. I have tried but I just can't go. I hate living in the dorm and sharing a bathroom—I've never had to do that before."

4. Identify specific questions that would explore the factors that may be affecting bowel elimination in this particular patient. Consider all the factors a new student may encounter in a new lifestyle at college.

Factor	Interview Question
Privacy	
Sufficient time	
Foods and fiber	
Dietary supplements	
Fluids	
Activity	

Factor	Interview Question
Medications	
Food allergy	
Food intolerances	

5. A rectal exam reveals that Sasha has a fecal impaction. The primary care provider orders a 90 mL oil-retention enema for Sasha. Discuss the procedure with Sasha to allay her anxiety and concerns.

_____

_____

_____

_____

_____

_____

_____

_____

_____

_____

_____

_____

_____

_____

_____

_____

_____

_____

_____

6. After an hour, Sasha reports that the enema was not successful. The primary care provider orders digital removal of the stool. How will you implement this treatment while minimizing Sasha's embarrassment and discomfort?

_____

_____

_____

_____

_____

_____

_____

_____

_____

_____

7. Upon discharge from the center, Sasha needs teaching on how to promote regular defecation. Discuss the key points that need to be taught to Sasha to ensure a healthy bowel routine.

_____

_____

_____

_____

_____

_____

_____

_____

_____

_____

Bowel Elimination: Diarrhea

Mr. Greaves is a direct admission from his assisted care facility to the intermediate care unit with dehydration secondary to profuse diarrhea. He is awake, alert, and oriented (×3, has a low-grade fever, abdominal cramps, and diarrhea (5 to 10 watery stools a day). He tells you, "I don't think I have gone this much in my entire life! I can't even describe how bad my bottom feels! I was just getting over my chest infection with all those antibiotic pills." You receive the following orders from the primary care provider:

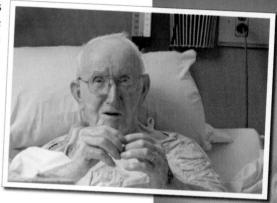

- Vital signs q4h while awake
- IV of lactated Ringer's solution (LR) @ 150 mL/hr
- BRAT diet
- Stool for occult blood, O&P, and *Clostridium difficile*
- BR/BRP with assistance
- Skin/wound care consult

1. Which order will you implement first? Why?

_____

_____

_____

2. You need to obtain a stool specimen for the ordered tests. Describe the process to complete this procedure considering Mr. Greaves's situation.

_____

_____

_____

_____

_____

3. The fecal occult blood test (FOBT) is done on the nursing unit. Describe the critical steps of this procedure that are necessary to ensure valid results.

_____

_____

_____

_____

_____

_____

_____

4. Mr. Greaves says to you, "I think I need some medication to stop this diarrhea. Could you ask the doctor for something?" How should you respond to this question?

_____

_____

_____

_____

_____

5. Mr. Greaves tells you, "I know this sounds crazy but I am hungry in spite of all this mess. What can you get me to eat?" Discuss the dietary order as you would for this patient.

_____

_____

_____

Sensory Perception

You have received a report on the new admission to your short-term rehabilitation unit. Mrs. Ida Henson is an 81-year-old female with left hemiplegia, left-side neglect, and left visual field deficit (homonymous hemianopsia) due to a stroke. She has a history of hypertension and insulin-dependent diabetes mellitus (IDDM), and she wears bilateral hearing aids.

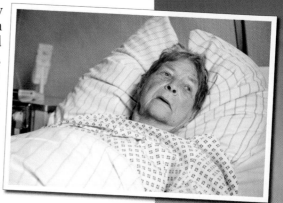

Prior to this event she was an extremely active octogenarian, working daily as a volunteer at the local botanical gardens, driving, and "supervising" the family. Her granddaughter lovingly states, "She likes being in the middle of controlled chaos; quiet makes her nervous. She would carry on a conversation with anyone—though I doubt she could ever hear half of it despite her hearing aids."

The transfer report includes the following nursing diagnoses for the plan of care:

- Disturbed sensory perception: auditory[†]
- Disturbed sensory perception: visual[†]

1. Discuss how this patient's medical problems have affected the reception and perception components of the sensory experience.

_____

_____

_____

_____

_____

_____

_____

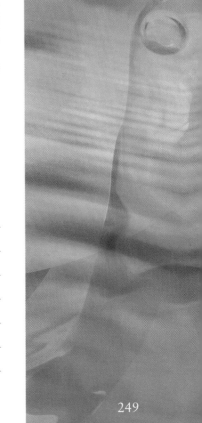

[†]© 2012 NANDA International

_____

_____

_____

_____

_____

2. Explore the potential impact of developmental variation and personality and lifestyle of this patient on sensory function.

Factor	Impact on Mrs. Henson's Sensory Function
Developmental	
Personality & lifestyle	

3. Based on your understanding of the admission information on this patient, list the defining characteristics that would support each of the identified nursing diagnoses.

_____

_____

_____

_____

4. Is this patient at greater risk for sensory overload or sensory deprivation? Give a rationale for your decision based on an understanding of the causes and patient characteristics and situation.

_____

_____

_____

_____

_____

_____

_____

5. Identify an appropriate NOC outcome and two individualized goals for this patient's nursing diagnoses.

After several weeks Mrs. Henson is progressing toward her goals for her stroke rehabilitation. However, the physical therapy assistant reports to you, "I don't know if it's just fatigue or what, but she doesn't seem to be hearing what I am telling her like she used to and I know she has her hearing aids in place."

6. What assessments should you initiate to explore this information given to you?

It is determined that Mrs. Henson has impacted cerumen. You receive an order for carbamide peroxide (Debrox) two drops each ear bid × 3 days, to be followed by otic irrigation on day four.

7. In this facility otic irrigations are done with a rubber bulb syringe. You delegate the otic irrigation to the licensed practical nurse (LPN). What steps should this nurse be able to verbalize to you to validate her competency in this procedure?

8. The LPN reports to you a good result from the irrigation but states, "Mrs. Henson sure is complaining of dizziness now." What does this indicate to you in your evaluation of the procedure? What remediation instruction should you give the LPN?

9. How will you evaluate successful outcomes for the otic irrigation for Mrs. Henson?

10. What generalized strategies can you put in place for the healthcare team to facilitate communication with Mrs. Henson in view of her hearing impairment and present health status?

Pain Management

Ms. Alanna Duffy, a nursing student is doing her preceptorship on the Nurses Improving Care for Healthsystem Elders (NICHE) dedicated medical unit. NICHE is a practice model for sensitive and exemplary care for all patients age 65 and older. NICHE supports the implementation of a variety of best practices, including prevention and management of pain (http://www.nicheprogram.org/niche_guiding_principles). Alanna has been assigned to care for the following patient:

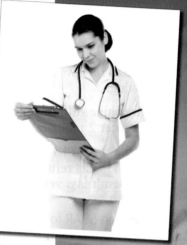

- Mr. Robert White, 73 years old, 2 days' post-operative for surgical decompression by laminectomy for cauda equina syndrome

    Mr. White rates his pain as a 10 and is very irritable, stating, "All this questioning is aggravating; you know I have pain—just give me what the doctor ordered as often as I can have it."

1. Formulate an appropriate response to this patient's statement.

_____

_____

_____

_____

_____

_____

2. Discuss the factors that may be influencing his pain experience. You may be creative in identifying potential issues for a patient with surgery as extensive as this with a projected long recovery. Mr. White is not used to being incapacitated and dependent on others.

_____

_____

Activity and Exercise

You have been assigned to care for Mr. Rich Tilly, a 32-year-old admitted to your short-term rehabilitation unit after a lengthy hospitalization following a bike crash that occurred during a triathlon competition. He had sustained a closed head injury resulting in a 14-day coma but is now awake, alert, and oriented. He also had fractures to the right femur and tibia and right radius. The leg fracture sites were stabilized with external fixation devices. He has a fiberglass cast on his right arm extending from his hand to his elbow. He can bend the right elbow. He is permitted no weight-bearing on the right leg. Goals of his rehabilitation include reconditioning and independence in mobility and self-care activities.

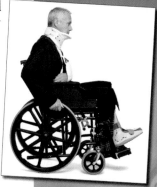

1. Due to the prolonged recovery from his head injury as well as musculoskeletal compromise, Mr. Tilly is at risk for the hazards of immobility. Discuss the system changes you should be looking for during the admission assessment. Include both a subjective (how would the patient verbalize the problem) and the objective measurements (physical assessment data) of the potential system effects. It may be helpful to reference the health assessment chapter of your textbook/laboratory book for normal and abnormal findings correlating to these system effects.

_____

_____

_____

_____

11. At the sixth week of his recovery, the cast on his right arm is removed after diagnostic radiology shows that the fracture to the right radius has fully healed. The wrist and hand joints are very stiff and weak, and he is encouraged to move them as much as possible. Describe the aspects of range of motion of those joints that you should teach Mr. Tilly to do to facilitate a full return of function in that extremity.

Joint	Range of Motion/Exercises
Wrist	
Hands/fingers	
Thumb	

12. Gaining strength in the arm has been a positive enforcer for his recovery. He asks you, "Why can't I have a pair of crutches instead of that walker to help me get around?" Using an SBAR format, how would you address this with the physiatrist?

S (Situation)	
B (Background)	
A (Assessment)	
R (Recommendations)	

13. Describe how you would teach Mr. Tilly to use crutches. What are the safety concerns you should address with him in the use of this modality?

_____

_____

_____

_____

_____

_____

_____

_____

_____

_____

_____

_____

_____

Sexual Health

As a cardiac rehabilitation nurse, you have been working with Mr. Fred Cavanaugh. He had an episode of sudden cardiac death due to dysrhythmias 2 months ago and received an implantable defibrillator. He is also taking amiodarone (Cordarone) to suppress ventricular irritability. He is progressing well in his rehabilitation. His wife accompanies him to all his visits to help facilitate success at home. Mr. Cavanaugh lovingly refers to his wife as "the warden," stating, "She keeps me in line but she will help me stay healthy. We've been together over 45 years. I couldn't do without her." In confidence Mrs. Cavanaugh discloses to you that her husband is worried about being unable "to perform."

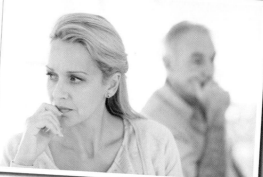

1. Discuss how you would explore Mrs. Cavanaugh's concerns using the guidelines for taking a sexual history.

_____

_____

_____

_____

_____

_____

_____

_____

_____

_____

_____

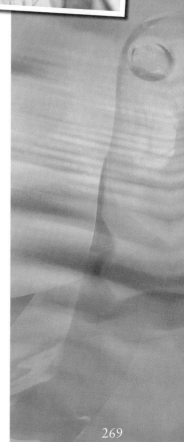

_____
_____
_____
_____

2. Formulate three open-ended questions to obtain more information regarding the nature of this concern. Examples:

_____
_____
_____
_____

In the history, Mrs. Cavanaugh tells you that her husband is still struggling with depression regarding his cardiac event and change in lifestyle. She tells you, "They have given him escitalopram [Lexapro] for it and it has helped him feel better about everything but still he isn't back to normal. I miss our close times."

3. Discuss the health and illness factors that may be affecting Mr. Cavanaugh's sexuality.

_____
_____
_____
_____
_____
_____
_____

4. You identify a nursing diagnosis of Sexual Dysfunction[†] related to altered body function with the NOC outcome being Sexual Functioning. Identify two individualized outcomes for Mr. Cavanaugh.

_____
_____

5. The suggested NIC intervention is sexual counseling. Formulate the dialogue you could initiate using the first two steps of the PLISSIT model (P-LI).

_____
_____
_____
_____
_____

_____

_____

_____

_____

_____

_____

_____

_____

During the counseling session, Mr. Cavanaugh states, "I never had any problems until this heart problem, and it got even worse when they started giving me this pill for my depression. What good is feeling better if it interferes with how I function?"

6. How would you respond to his concern?

_____

_____

_____

_____

7. Using the SBAR format, how would you communicate this concern to the primary care provider?

S (Situation)	
B (Background)	
A (Assessment)	
R (Recommendations)	

8. The primary care provider orders a trial of sildenafil (Viagra) for Mr. Cavanaugh. Discuss the patient teaching that needs to be completed in regard to facilitating a normal sexual response.

_____

_____

_____

_____

A physical therapist assistant student has been shadowing you at the cardiac rehabilitation center. She says to you, "I thought once you got old, sex wasn't really a concern anymore."

9. How would you address this comment from an understanding of developmental stage in aging adults?

_____

_____

_____

_____

_____

In addition she says, "I would be hesitant to discuss this kind of stuff with patients. How do you handle some of the off-color comments that are often expressed? I know it's more insecurity than personal but it would really upset me."

10. What would you tell this student in regard to dealing with inappropriate sexual behavior that may be encountered in a healthcare setting?

_____

_____

_____

_____

_____

Sleep and Rest

This week in clinical Damita is assigned to care for Mr. Henry McAllister, who is recovering from an acute myocardial infarction (MI). It was found that severe sleep apnea contributed to his cardiac event. He is recovering well from his MI but is now on a CPAP machine at night to help with his sleep apnea. The CPAP treatment requires that a snug-fitting mask be worn over the nose and mouth during the night. The patient has found it difficult to get used to wearing the mask. Damita visits the patient the evening of her clinical preparation and the patient tells her, "I don't think I am ever going to get any sleep wearing this thing. I am so drowsy during the day and I can't even think straight. I am so overwhelmingly tired. I feel like I am going to suffocate even though I know it is helping me. It's hard enough to get any rest in the hospital without adding this to it all. I miss the simple things that helped me to sleep at night like my music and my air conditioner running."

1. What did the patient mean by "It's hard enough to get any rest in the hospital"?

_____

_____

_____

_____

_____

_____

_____

_____

2. What data from this short interaction validate a nursing diagnosis of Disturbed Sleep Pattern?[†]

_____

_____

_____

3. In addition, the patients tells Damita, "I know that I had a pretty big heart attack but ever since I've gotten treatment I been having weird dreams—almost like nightmares." How should Damita explore this comment? What could be the potential etiology of this aspect of the patient's insomnia?

_____

_____

_____

_____

_____

_____

_____

_____

In preparation for her clinical day, Damita develops a plan of care to facilitate restful sleep for this patient. She identifies the following nursing interventions to promote sleep:

- Sleep Enhancement
- Environmental Management: Comfort

4. For each of the following interventions used to promote sleep, write a nursing action that individualizes it to this patient's care situation:

_____

_____

_____

_____

_____

_____

_____

_____

_____

_____

_____

5. She adds to the interventions "back massage daily at HS." Considering this patient's status, is this an appropriate intervention at this time? Why or why not?

_____

_____

_____

_____

_____

_____

6. The patient inquires about the possibility of "getting a pill to help me sleep." Using the SBAR format, construct the dialogue for use with the primary care provider. Consider all the data Damita has collected regarding the patient's history/experience of MI and from her conversation with the patient the evening of her preparation work.

S (Situation)	
B (Background)	
A (Assessment)	
R (Recommendations)	

7. How can Damita best measure the quality of sleep for this patient after implementation of the nursing interventions?

_____

_____

Skin Integrity

Marya, a first-semester nursing student, will be doing a rotation with Francis Obermyer, RN CWCN, one of the nurses on the wound care team at the hospital. Francis is a certified wound care nurse. In preparation for the rotation she was provided with the following census printout for some of the patients that Francis will be rounding on the following day. Marya will have the opportunity to do wound assessments as well as the indicated interventions for wound care.

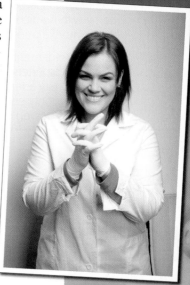

Patient	Primary & Secondary Medical Diagnoses	Age	Wound Type	Dressing Type	Treatment Orders
A	Diabetic ketoacidosis; renal insufficiency, diabetic neuropathy	74	Diabetic foot ulcer, left great toe (arterial ulcer)	Gauze	Wet-to-moist saline dressing bid
B	Deep vein thrombosis (DVT), right leg, peripheral vascular disease, hypertension	58	Venous stasis ulcer, left lateral malleous	Alginate	Alginate dressing daily Irrigate wound with NSS with each dressing change
C	Colon cancer, s/p exploratory laparotomy with hemicolectomy, morbid obesity	49	Surgical incision with staples	Gauze Penrose drain	Advance Penrose drain 6 mm daily
D	Urosepsis, dementia, cachexia, hypertension, coronary artery disease, incontinence (bladder & bowel)	92	Pressure ulcer (coccyx)	New admission—to be determined	

1. For each of the patients, discuss the factors that could be affecting their skin integrity.

Factors	Impact on Skin Integrity	Patient(s) Affected
Age-related		
Mobility		
Nutrition/hydration		

Factors	Impact on Skin Integrity	Patient(s) Affected
Sensation/cognition		
Circulation		
Medications		
Moisture on skin		
Fever		
Contamination/ infection		
Lifestyle		

2. For the first three patients, what are the expected characteristics of the type of wound for each that the student can anticipate finding when the dressings are changed during the day's rounds?

Patient	Wound type	Expected Findings
A	Diabetic foot ulcer, left great toe (arterial)	
B	Venous stasis ulcer, left lateral malleous	
C	Surgical incision with staples	

3. Explain why the dressing ordered for each wound is appropriate to the situation.

Wound Type	Dressing	Rationale for Ordered Dressing
Diabetic foot ulcer, left great toe (arterial)	Gauze	
Venous stasis ulcer, left lateral malleous	Alginate	
Surgical incision with staples	Gauze	

4. How will Marya know what/how much dressing materials will be needed for each type of dressing?

_____

_____

_____

_____

_____

5. When planning for implementation of these wound care procedures, what are the commonalities of procedural steps in readying the patients for the dressing change?

_____

_____

_____

_____

6. Marya plans to use a gown and face shield for each of the ordered treatments. Is doing so appropriate to the procedures? Give a rationale for your decision.

_____

_____

_____

_____

The day's rounds begin with a visit to the post-operative patient. The dressing needs to be changed and the Penrose drain advanced 6 mm per physician orders. This is the first time that the Penrose drain order will be implemented.

7. What equipment will be needed to implement the order?

_____

_____

8. The patient has Montgomery straps holding the dressings covering the Penrose drain. What is the purpose of these straps?

_____

_____

9. The patient is extremely apprehensive about "anyone pulling on something sticking out of me." Describe how Marya should explain the procedure to the patient.

_____

_____

_____

_____

_____

_____

_____

The next dressing procedure involves irrigation of the wound and placement of the alginate dressing.

10. How should the patient be positioned to complete the irrigation?

_____

_____

18. The NOC outcome of Wound Healing, Secondary Intention is chosen and the NIC interventions address pressure ulcer care. In review of the individualized interventions appropriate to this problem, which interventions can be delegated to the unlicensed assistive personnel?

_____

_____

_____

_____

_____

Oxygenation

The senior students are participating in an outreach program to enhance the pulmonary health of the community. They are involved in two aspects of the program, prevention/teaching, and symptom surveillance and diagnostic testing for infectious pulmonary diseases with referral as indicated.

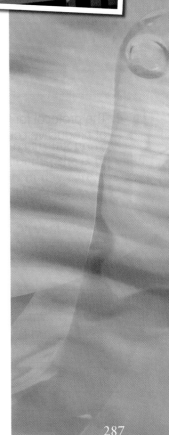

In preparation for their work the instructor asks them to study the following entities in pulmonary disease: upper respiratory infection, influenza, pneumonia, and tuberculosis. The common pathological processes in these diseases include inflammation, infection, production of secretions, and compromised oxygenation.

Every person visiting the program has the following assessments done:

- Health history: assessment of risk factors inclusive of any smoking history
- Vital signs and pulse oximetry
- Pulmonary assessment: breathing pattern/effort, lung sounds, and presence/absence of cough

1. The nurse at the outreach program says to the students, "We get a lot of older adults coming for appointments; they have developmental changes that put them at risk for many pulmonary problems." Discuss what the nurse meant by this statement.

14. The respiratory therapy technician comes in to do chest physiotherapy with Mr. King. To best clear the secretions from the middle and lower lobes of his right lung, what positions should be used to facilitate success of secretion mobilization and removal?

_____

15. The primary diagnosis for Mr. King is Impaired gas exchange† related to alveolar-capillary membrane changes secondary to inflammation and infection. The NOC outcome is Respiratory Status: Gas Exchange. Individualize patient outcomes for Mr. King.

_____

_____

_____

_____

_____

16. Mr. King asks the nurse for "help staying away from cigarettes when I get home." Using an SBAR format, how should the nurse address this issue with the primary care provider?

S (Situation)	
B (Background)	
A (Assessment)	
R (Recommendations)	

Perfusion

■ Mr. Theodore Jeffers is a 73-year-old admitted to the pro-
gressive coronary care unit with a diagnosis of atypical chest
pain and congestive heart failure. He has a history of acute
myocardial infarction, deep vein thrombosis, hypertension,
diabetes mellitus, and gouty arthritis. He reports "spasm-
like" chest pain over his breastbone and difficulty "catching
my breath." His admission data includes the following:

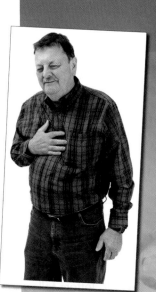

- Chest pain rated as a 4 on a scale of 1 to 10; states,
  "It feels like my heart is clenching like a fist—I am not
  sure I can call it pain."
- BP: 172/100 – 102 – 30
- Temperature: 99.2°F
- O$_2$ saturation: 90% on room air
- Lungs: fine crackles throughout all lung fields
- Heart sounds with S$_3$ present
- 4+ pitting edema, decreased peripheral pulses bilaterally,
  feet cool to touch
- Height: 72 inches; Weight: 231#; BMI: 31.3

1. Mr. Jeffers is placed on continuous cardiac monitoring. As the
   primary nurse, what are your responsibilities in the care of a
   patient requiring this type of monitoring?

Fluid, Electrolyte, and Acid-Base Balance

As a senior student you are assigned to work with a preceptor in the Emergency Department. It is a very busy day and it seems as if every patient, regardless of chief complaint, has an issue with fluid, electrolyte, and/or acid-base balance.

The first patient you see is a 37-year-old landscaper who is brought to the ED after collapsing on a job at the local country club. He is slightly confused but is able to tell you he feels dizzy and weak. His skin is flushed, dry, and with poor turgor. He has dry, sticky mucous membranes. The nurse identifies a nursing diagnosis of deficient fluid volume.

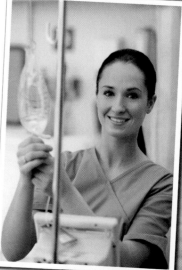

1. Describe how each of the following would change and the rationale for the change in the presence of deficient fluid volume:
   • Heart rate
   • Blood pressure
   • Serum hematocrit
   • Urinary output
   • Urine specific gravity
   • Weight

Parameter	Expected Change	Rationale
Heart rate		
Blood pressure		
Serum hematocrit		
Urinary output		
Urine specific gravity		
Weight		

2. What is usually the first indicator that an individual needs more fluids?

_____

3. The ED physician orders IV fluids for this patient. What types of fluids are indicated for a fluid volume deficit due to dehydration?

_____

_____

_____

   The preceptor tells you to go ahead and initiate an IV site and start the fluids. The fluid order is to start 1000 mL of fluid as ordered at 150 mL/hr. The infusion tubing has a drop factor of 15 gtt/mL.

4. This infusion will run by gravity rather than an infusion pump. How many drops per minute should you time the infusion at to ensure the correct hourly rate?

5. What factors should you be concerned about that may compromise the gravity infusion rate? How will you intervene for these factors?

Factor	Nursing Action

6. The patient has a "full sleeve" tattoo on both arms. Discuss the implications of this finding and how you will initiate the intravenous site.

_____

_____

_____

_____

_____

_____

7. You have difficulty finding a vein in the presence of the deficient fluid volume. What strategies can you employ to help make a vein more visible/palpable?

_____

_____

_____

_____

_____

_____

8. Considering the diagnosis, patient presentation, and fluid orders, what size catheter is indicated in this situation? Give a rationale for your choice.

_____

_____

_____

_____

9. After 30 minutes of the infusion, the patient states, "My arm where the needle is feels funny." What should you do first? What further data do you need from the patient?

_____

_____

_____

_____

_____

_____

_____

_____

_____

_____

Several hours later the patient is feeling better and is now oriented × 3. The ED physician wants the patient to be drinking oral fluids without difficulty prior to being discharged from the ED.

10. Discuss the strategies to increase fluid intake that are most appropriate to this setting.

_____

_____

_____

_____

11. The patient is discharged after adequate hydration. Discharge teaching includes ways to prevent this from happening again on the job. What key points should the nurse include in the teaching applicable to the job site?

_____

_____

_____

_____

The next patient is a 67-year-old patient who presents with a chief complaint: "I can't sleep at night—I can't lie down, I get so out of breath." She is sitting in high Fowler's position on the exam table. She has a history of heart problems. She is diagnosed with acute exacerbation of congestive heart failure, and you identify a nursing diagnosis of Fluid Volume Excess (FVE).[†]

12. What is the term you should use to document the patient's chief complaint regarding her breathing?

_____

_____

13. Besides the respiratory difficulty exhibited by the patient, what manifestation of FVE may be immediately visible on assessment?

_____

_____

_____

_____

The physician gives the following orders: (You may need to review your drug resources to help you understand the medication orders.)

- D_5LR at 100 mL/hr
- Use infusion pump
- Furosemide (Lasix) 80 mg IV now
- Potassium citrate (K-Lyte) 10 mEq orally now and q4h × 2 doses
- O_2 2–5 LPM to keep O_2 sat greater than 92%

14. Which order should the nurse question? Why?

_____

_____

_____

_____

_____

15. Over the course of 4 hours the patient has a weight loss of 11 pounds. This represents how much fluid loss?

_____

_____

The patient was admitted to the facility and after 2 days is ready for discharge. Discharge orders include a low-sodium (2000 mg/day) diet and a fluid restriction of 1500 mL/day.

16. Describe the key information that the patient needs to know to follow these instructions.

_____

_____

_____

_____

_____

_____

_____

_____

_____

_____

_____

_____

_____

Another patient is brought to the Emergency Department by a neighbor who noticed her sitting, confused, on her front steps. The patient is a 24-year-old female and unable to give a valid history at this time. Admission data include the following:

- Neurological: Confused
- Pulmonary: Respirations 28 breaths/min and shallow, lungs clear
- Cardiovascular: Irregular rapid pulse, ECG shows flattened T waves
- Gastrointestinal: Hypoactive bowel sounds
- Musculoskeletal: Muscle weakness

17. The preceptor identifies a nursing diagnosis of Risk for decreased cardiac output[†] related to electrolyte imbalance. What is the electrolyte imbalance that is being presented by this patient?

_____

18. What is the specific NOC outcome for this electrolyte imbalance? Identify two expected outcomes for this patient.

_____

_____

_____

19. In light of the patient's confusion, what medication order can you anticipate from the ED physician to correct this electrolyte problem? What are your responsibilities in the implementation of the orders?

_____

_____

_____

_____

_____

_____

Due to a bed shortage, the patient remains in the ED for treatment for the next 12 hours. At that time her confusion has cleared and her apical pulse is now regular though still somewhat tachycardic at 102 beats/min. She tells you that she had been using her grandmother's "water pills" to help her lose weight.

20. What is the significance of this information?

21. It is decided to discharge her home with instructions regarding dietary intake to ensure good serum levels of the compromised electrolyte. What foods should be included in these instructions?

A patient presents to the ED a diagnosis of exacerbation of Crohn's disease with malabsorption syndrome. He is also severely dehydrated from the excessive diarrhea associated with the disease. A concurrent concern is hypocalcemia.

22. What subjective data would you expect to gain from the patient that describe symptoms of hypocalcemia?

23. Describe how you would assess for hypocalcemia in this setting.

24. Your preceptor tells you, "Keep an eye on his breathing, okay?" What is the significance of this directive?

Hospitalization is required for this patient for stabilization and treatment of both the hypocalcemia and the exacerbation of his disease. At discharge orders, include oral calcium supplements and/or a diet high in calcium.

25. What is the best dietary source of calcium? What additional dietary supplement is necessary for adequate calcium absorption?

26. Discuss alternative dietary choices for the patient who states, "I don't like milk products. I am lactose intolerant."

The last patient you see today presents to the ED with a complaint of chest tightness, tingling in the hands, and headache. He has noticeable trembling of the hands. He tells you, "I swear I think I am having a heart attack!" His vital signs are BP 162/88 – 104 – 32 and afebrile. The ED physician orders laboratory work including cardiac panel, chemistry panel, CBC, and arterial blood gases (ABGs). He tells you "I think he is having an anxiety attack."

27. What would you anticipate the ABG results to be (disorder and values) if this diagnosis is correct?

28. What is the most appropriate nursing diagnosis, NOC outcome, and NIC intervention for this acid-base disorder?

29. How would you assist the patient to compensate for this acid-base disorder?

Nursing Functions

Leading and Management

Hillary Hockenberry has been a nurse for 4 years in a long-term care facility. Recently, the position of unit manager has become available and she is considering applying for it. Peers have encouraged her to consider doing so and have commented, "You are a born leader and manager and will do really well in the position." Hillary Hockenberry is now asking herself the following questions:

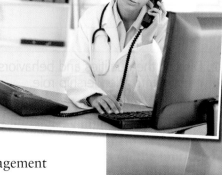

- Am I ready for a position like this?
- What management skills will I need to be a good unit manager?
- What are the rewards and challenges to a management position?

She seeks input from both the former unit manager, who is now the assistant director of nursing (ADON), whom she views as a mentor, as well as the preceptor whom she originally worked with as a new graduate.

After several months, conflict has arisen between the UAP of the skilled care unit and those on the custodial care/assisted living unit regarding feeding responsibilities during the meals. The UAP are very territorial regarding "their" residents and do not feel that they should have to assist other residents in the dining room since "their people" are there to help them. Due to the higher acuity of the skilled unit residents, they require more assistance with feeding than those who are more independent from the custodial/assisted living unit. The UAP from the assisted living unit feel that they should not have to "pick up the slack" with feeding needs of the residents from the other unit. As the unit manager, Hillary needs to resolve this conflict for optimal resident outcomes.

12. Using the steps of conflict resolution, how should the unit manager work through this problem?

_____

_____

- Identify the problem
- Generate possible solutions
- Evaluate suggested solutions
- Choose the best solution
- Implement the solution
- Evaluate—is the problem resolved?

Identify the problem	
Generate possible solutions	
Evaluate suggested solutions	
Choose the best solution	
Implement the solution	
Evaluate—is the problem resolved?	

13. Discuss how time management may be an important component in the integration of the dining process when one staff member says, "I can't help feed residents when all I can think about is that I have to administer medications and complete the treatments on my 30 residents." Consider the suggestions for time management. Discuss which ones may be helpful in this situation.

Informatics

A new nurse is being oriented to the clinic's computer system that includes the electronic health records as well as support programs that provide information needed in clinical decision-making. Examples include medication/pharmacology information, standardized nursing languages, and search engines for finding and validating best practices for nursing. It also provides an avenue for communication via electronic mail and synchronous modes with other users of the system. One of the members of the class remarks, "This is

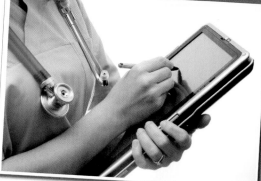

great—instead of 'paint by numbers' I have 'patient care by numbers.' All this information tells us exactly what, when, and how to do our job."

1. Dispute this statement using the definition and elements of informatics as well as how these elements are integrative to the use of the nursing process.

_____

_____

_____

_____

_____

_____

2. Computers provide many avenues for communication within the context of nursing practice. The uses of these modalities are limited only by your imagination. For each of the types of electronic communication, list how this new nurse (and yourself as a nursing student) could use these methods to enhance your education and your practice. Be creative—some of

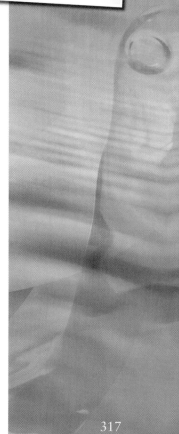

the uses may already be in place or you may very well design a new use for it within the profession.
• Electronic mail
• Text messaging
• Web conferencing
• Webinars
• Electronic mail (Listserv)
• Social networking
• Telehealth

Modality	Example of Present Use	Potential Uses: Practice/ Education
Electronic mail		
Text messaging		
Web conferencing		
Webinars		
Electron mail list (Listserv)		
Social networking		
Telehealth		

After being trained on the computer system, the new graduate is using the system to update a patient's EHR with data gathered during a follow-up clinic visit for a previously diagnosed viral infection. The patient asks the nurse, "Does all this computer work make your life easier or more complicated? I worry about people getting to my records—you know you hear all this stuff about people hacking into government systems."

3. Based on the benefits and ethical use of EHRs, give an appropriate response to this patient's concerns.

The patient further tells the nurse, "I really like my computer at home because there is so much information on it. I feel like I have a second doctor whenever I need one. In fact, I came across some great information on how to get rid of this infection after the doctor decided I didn't need a prescription at the last visit." The patient gives the nurse a printout from a Web site recommending colloidal silver as a home remedy for viral infections.

4. What simple instruction should the nurse give this patient regarding the credibility of Web sites?

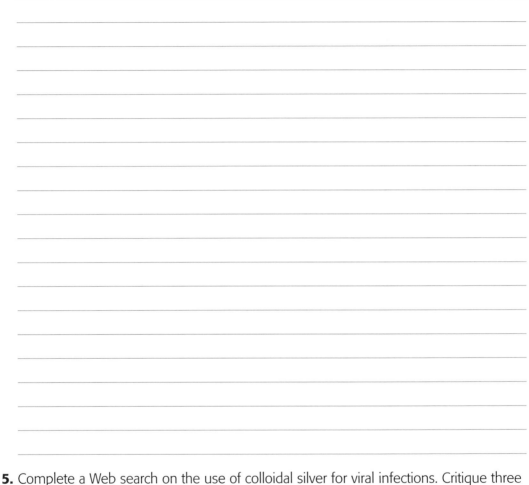

5. Complete a Web search on the use of colloidal silver for viral infections. Critique three sites for the following characteristics:
- Authority
- Currency
- Purpose
- Content quality

Site	Authority	Currency	Purpose	Content

6. Summarize your perspective on the authenticity of information found regarding this topic. How would you best use this information in your clinical decision-making?

_____

_____

_____

_____

_____

_____

Holism

Dr. Dale, a university professor, is a 67-year-old man in for his annual examination. He has no medical issues but mentions to the nurse that he feels he doesn't sleep as well as he could. He states that he usually goes to bed around 2100, sleeps only about 2 to 3 hours at a time, and is usually up by 0400 each morning. The nighttime awakenings are described as "abrupt," and he says he must work to "put myself back to sleep." Although the quantity of sleep seems sufficient for him, he verbalizes the desire for "more peaceful and longer" sleep. In the past he has tried prescriptive sleep aids but had unpleasant effects including disorientation and sluggishness. He runs 8 miles each morning and participates in a yoga class two evenings a week. The yoga instructor suggested exploring complementary and alternative modalities (CAM) and a more holistic approach for self-care.

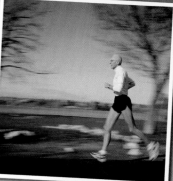

1. Does Dr. Dale fit the composite of a patient who would use CAM? Why or why not?

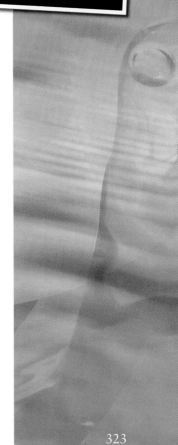

For this patient, the nurse identifies the following diagnoses: Readiness for enhanced sleep.[†]

2. From the situation, identify the defining characteristics that validate this diagnosis for this patient.

_____

_____

_____

3. Identify two NOC outcomes for the diagnosis.

_____

_____

_____

_____

4. What is the major intervention pertinent to the outcomes that link well with holistic care?

_____

Dr. Dale agrees with the diagnosis and states a desire to find therapy/therapies that best integrate with his lifestyle and his own philosophy of self-driven wellness. He states, "I don't want any of that touchy-feely stuff or needles put everywhere." He recognizes the need for traditional medicine but wants interventions that address all spheres of humanness: physical, emotional, cultural, and spiritual.

5. Which two categories of healing modalities would best fit with this patient's life perspective? Explain your choices.

_____

_____

_____

_____

_____

_____

_____

_____

_____

_____

_____

_____

6. Describe to Dr. Dale each of the different interventions listed under the two healing modalities previously identified and how they might be used to enhance sleep.

Choose three interventions that would be applicable for this patient situation. Give a rationale for each one of your chosen interventions.

_____

_____

_____

_____

_____

_____

_____

_____

_____

7. The patient asks you, "Do you believe in these therapies or use them yourself?" Based on your own life situation how would you respond to this question and best support these interventions for the patient?

_____

_____

_____

_____

_____

_____

_____

_____

Health Promotion

A group of students in a nursing research course have been working in a concurrent course with geriatric patients at a local independent-living senior center. The individuals whom they have been interacting with are active seniors but have indicated a desire to "feel better" and be "more active."

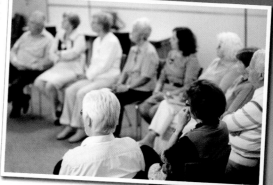

1. Does this situation represent health promotion or health protection? Why?

_____

_____

_____

_____

_____

_____

_____

2. What level of prevention would be represented by programs to meet these desired outcomes?

_____

_____

_____

_____

_____

As part of a research project, the students have decided to implement a program of wellness to see if it meets the needs of this group of individuals. The center is supportive of introducing modalities to promote wellness in this population.

3. Using Pender's Health Promotion Model, what could be the group's perceived benefits of action (positive or reinforcing consequences of undertaking a health behavior) as well as perceived barriers to action (perceptions of blocks, hurdles, and personal costs of undertaking a health behavior) within this setting?

_____

_____

_____

_____

_____

_____

_____

_____

_____

_____

_____

_____

4. What types of health promotion programs (the intervention) could be implemented in this setting? Give examples of what your group could do within the identified types that will address the issue to "feel better" and be "more active."

_____

_____

_____

_____

_____

_____

_____

_____

_____

_____

5. Describe the parts of a health promotion assessment.

Component	Description/Pertinence to a Wellness Program
Health history	
Physical examination	
Fitness assessment	
Lifestyle/risk appraisal	
Stress review	
Analysis of health beliefs	
Nutritional assessment	
Screening activities	

6. For this group of participants, the majority of information can be found in their EHR associated with the facility. Rank (1 being the greatest and 8 being the least) the pertinence of the information to the development and implementation of a flexibility and balance program (changing lifestyle and behavior) that will be the first step in a comprehensive activity program for this group. Give a rationale for how you ranked the components.

Component	Rank	Rationale
Health history		
Physical examination		
Fitness assessment		
Lifestyle/risk appraisal		
Stress review		
Analysis of health beliefs		
Nutritional assessment		
Screening activities		

7. Identify two wellness diagnoses and an NOC standardized outcome with a specific participant outcome for each diagnosis.

_____

_____

_____

_____

_____

_____

_____

_____

8. Provide a generalized NIC wellness intervention for each diagnosis.

_____

_____

_____

_____

_____

_____

_____

_____

9. Discuss how role modeling, providing health education, and providing and facilitating support for lifestyle change can each be implemented to meet the desired outcomes for this group.

Strategy	Implementation
Role modeling	
Health education	
Support for lifestyle change	

Context for Nurses' Work

Perioperative Nursing

Mr. Bane Ka'uhane is a 66-year-old male admitted to the surgical unit with a diagnosis of abdominal mass. He has been complaining of vague symptoms for the past 3 months. These symptoms include intermittent indigestion, abdominal pain, and constipation. His medical history includes COPD, PVD, and insulin-dependent diabetes mellitus. He takes the following medications at home:

• Prednisone (Sterapred) 10 mg PO daily
• Insulin glargine (Lantus) 24 units SQ at 2200
• Ipratropium (Atrovent) inhaler 2 puffs QID
• ASA (Ecotrin) 81 mg PO daily

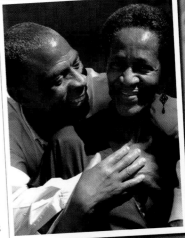

The nursing assessment/history done on admission includes the following data:
  Objective data:

• Wt/Ht: 213#   70 inches
• VS: BP 140/88 – 84 – 20 – 97.8
• Lungs: clear with intermittent expiratory wheeze
                left lower base

- CV: HR 84 beats/min and regular weak dorsalis pedis pulses bilaterally, skin warm and dry, feet cool to touch
- GI: Abdomen round, distended, active bowel sounds
- GU: Voids adequate amounts of clear yellow urine
- Allergy: Betadine

Subjective:

- "I'm coming in to find out what's going on in my belly."
- "I'm sure it's something fixable."
- "I don't want my wife to worry about me; I am not sure she is going to be able to handle all of this."
- "I keep my sugar pretty well normal. My breathing problems give me more trouble."

Mr. Ka'uhane is scheduled for an exploratory laparotomy at 0800 in the morning. His preoperative orders include:

- Labs: CBC with differential and a comprehensive metabolic panel
- NPO at 0600 and begin IV of 1000 NS at 50 mL/hr
- Prep abdomen with Phisohex scrub × 3. Cover abdomen with sterile towel after prep completed
- Have permit signed: I have discussed the surgical procedure/risks/expectations/outcomes
- Consult Pulmonary Services, re: Respiratory status
- Pre-op medications:
  - Atropine 0.4 mg with Demerol 50 mg IM on call to OR
  - Nembutal 25 mg IM on call to OR

1. In reviewing Mr. Ka'uhane's orders, which order should be questioned by the nurse?

_____

_____

_____

_____

2. Based on knowledge of his underlying medical problems and risks associated with age, how could these problems and risks affect the perioperative experience?

_____

_____

_____

_____

_____

_____

_____

3. How might Mr. Ka'uhane's routine meds place him at a higher surgical risk?

_____

_____

_____

_____

_____

_____

4. Based on the subjective data, identify the priority nursing diagnosis to meet the psychosocial needs of Mr. and Mrs. Ka'uhane.

_____

_____

5. You are completing pre-operative teaching regarding the routine nursing measures that Mr. and Mrs. Ka'uhane can expect during the post-operative period. How should you respond to the following questions? (You may need to review what an exploratory laparotomy is to help with this answer.)

_____

_____

_____

_____

_____

_____

_____

_____

_____

_____

_____

_____

_____

6. You are completing the pre-operative checklist. What is the last clinical procedure to be completed before administration of the pre-op medications?

_____

_____

_____

7. What physiological effects can you anticipate secondary to the pre-op medications?

_____

_____

_____

_____

Mr. Ka'uhane is transferred to the OR table and readied for surgery.

8. Discuss the importance of the Patient Safety Goals and the World Health Organization's (WHO) Surgical Safety Checklist in preventing mistakes in surgery.

_____

_____

_____

_____

_____

_____

_____

_____

_____

_____

_____

_____

_____

Mr. Ka'uhane has completed surgery and is transferred to the PACU. His present status is:

- Extremely drowsy but arousable
- Respirations 14/min and regular and deep, on 40% face tent, O_2 sat 94%
- Skin cool and dry, color pale
- Cardiac monitor: normal cardiac rhythm, no irregular beats
- Abdomen: midline dressing dry and intact
- Jackson-Pratt drainage device with moderate amount of bloody drainage
- NG tube to LWS of brownish/clear gastric drainage
- No bowel sounds present
- Foley to BSD of 60–100 mL/hr, light-yellow urine
- IV therapy
  - #1: 1000 mL LR at 100 mL/hr
  - #2: 1000 D5 1/2 NS with 20 units of regular insulin at 50 mL/hr

He had an uneventful surgery and the mass was removed without incidence. The OR nurse reports that Mr. Ka'uhane had a total of 4200 mL of IV fluids and a urinary output of 2700. Estimated blood loss was 525 mL. He did not require blood replacement. The abdominal incision was closed with staples and retention sutures and the dressing is dry and intact. Vital signs remained stable throughout the procedure.

9. He received general anesthesia throughout the procedure. The PACU nurse should assess for what frequent complaints related to this type of anesthesia?

10. In light of Mr Ka'uhane's medical history, how might the anesthesia contribute to the development of post-operative complications?

11. In reviewing the data above, which data, if any, need to be brought to the attention of the surgeon?

12. Identify the sites most at risk for pressure compromise secondary to surgical positioning.

Mr. Ka'uhane remained stable in the PACU. His vital signs are stable, his urinary output is adequate, and he is exhibiting no signs/symptoms of hypo/hyperglycemia. He is discharged to the surgical unit. His postoperative orders include:

- Vital signs q1h × 4, then q2h × 4, then q4h if stable
- NG tube to low intermittent suction, irrigate q2h with 30 mL NSS
- NPO, I&O q4h
- O_2 4 L/min nasal cannula, keep sats greater than 94%
- HHN Proventil 0.25 mg with 2 mL NSS q6h
- Incentive spirometry q1h while awake
- Foley to BSD
- IV D5 ¼ NS at 125 mL/hr
- OOB to chair this evening
- SCDs
- May change dressing prn, begin in AM after surgical rounds
- Medications:
  - Sliding scale insulin per protocol
  - Morphine 2 mg IV q2h prn for moderate pain less than 7
  - Morphine 4 mg IV q2h prn for severe pain equal to or greater than 7
  - Zofran 4 mg IV q4h prn nausea
  - Lovenox 40 mg SQ daily

13. Based on knowledge of client condition and surgical procedure, what is the number one priority for Mr. Ka'uhane during the post-operative phase of his experience?

_____

_____

_____

_____

14. How can nursing help with Mrs. Ka'uhane's role as facilitator of Mr. Ka'uhane's recovery?

_____

_____

_____

_____

_____

15. The nurse aide taking Mr. Ka'uhane's vital signs reports to you that Mrs. Ka'uhane is very upset over how often they are being done and verbalized that "something must be wrong!" How would you respond to Mrs. Ka'uhane?

_____

_____

_____

_____

16. The sequential compression device is in place when you receive Mr. Ka'uhane from the PACU. How will you check for proper fit to eliminate excess pressure and overcompression?

_____

_____

_____

17. You note that there is a small amount of drainage on the surgical dressing. The order reads that it is not to be changed prior to morning rounds. What is the appropriate action in this situation?

_____

_____

_____

_____

_____

_____

_____

_____

18. You tell your preceptor that you are familiar with the policy of the NG irrigation procedure but that you have never done it. She offers to demonstrate it to you. Before completing this procedure she checks for bowel sounds and documents active bowel sounds × 4 quadrants as she can hear intermittent rhythmic "whooshing" upon auscultation. Prior to instilling the irrigant into the nasogastric tube she disconnects the NG tube from the suction source, pulls up the ordered amount of NSS and instills it into the tube using the piston action of the syringe. After this she reconnects the tubing to the suction source telling you, "It's pretty simple." Critique the steps of the assessment and procedure as you saw it done. What would you do differently, if anything? Give a rationale.

_____

_____

_____

_____

_____

_____

_____

_____

_____

_____

_____

_____

19. In using his flow-oriented incentive spirometry Mr. Ka'uhane is proud that he is able to take brisk low-volume breaths that snap the balls to the top of the chamber. What is the appropriate response to his use of the IS?

_____

_____

_____

_____

_____

_____

20. Based on Mr. Ka'uhane's history and present assessment data, he is at high risk for which major post-operative complication(s)? Give a rationale for the choices that you made. Identify collaborative interventions (interdisciplinary) that can help prevent these complications

Complication	At Risk	Rationale	Interventions
Aspiration pneumonia			
Atelectasis			
Pneumonia			
Pulmonary embolus			
Thrombophlebitis			

Complication	At Risk	Rationale	Interventions
Hypovolemia			
Hemorrhage			
Nausea/vomiting			
Abdominal distention			
Constipation			
Ileus			
Renal failure			
Urinary retention			
Urinary tract infection			
Dehiscence			
Evisceration			
Wound infection			

Community-Based Care

As part of an introduction to the many career roles within the nursing profession, Javier Rivera-Sanchez is assigned to shadow a nurse from the county health department. The county demographics portray an aggregate at increased risk of adverse health outcomes as evidenced by a high percentage of elderly members of Asian descent. This vulnerable population was identified through review of statistics that indicated a high incidence of hospital admissions due to hip fracture secondary to osteoporosis with subsequent physiological compromise requiring the use of complex community resources.

1. In review of *Healthy People 2020*, specifically related to osteoporosis (overview, objectives, interventions) identify the objectives and interventions for osteoporosis. (http://www.healthypeople.gov/2020/topicsobjectives2020/overview.aspx?topicId=3)

_____

_____

_____

_____

_____

_____

_____

_____

2. Discuss how the threefold services of community-based care—community health, public health nursing, and community-oriented nursing—are necessary to the success of outcomes for this 2020 topic.

_____

_____

_____

_____

_____

_____

_____

_____

_____

_____

_____

_____

_____

_____

_____

_____

_____

_____

_____

3. Describe possible community nursing interventions for this issue using the classification system of primary, secondary, and tertiary levels of care.

_____

_____

_____

_____

_____

_____

_____

_____

_____

_____

The health department has identified that inadequate nutritional intake of calcium and vitamin D, a sedentary lifestyle, and genetic factors related to biological variation found in this ethnic group to be related to the incidence of osteoporosis in this aggregate. Using the Omaha System (http://www.omahasystem.org/) and the problem classification scheme, the following domain and problems were identified:

- Domain: Health Related Behaviors
- Problem Classification Schemes: Nutrition, Physical Activity
- Problem modifiers:

_____

_____

4. Identify the two appropriate diagnostic statements that address the osteoporosis issue in this community using the Omaha Problem Classification Scheme.

_____

_____

5. For each of the diagnostic statements, create expected outcomes using the Omaha Problem Rating Scale.

Health Promotion in Group Nutrition

Concept	Present Status	Expected Outcome

Health Promotion in Group Physical Activity

Concept	Present Status	Expected Outcome

6. Using the Omaha taxonomy, write two nursing interventions in the format of category + target for each of the nursing diagnoses you identified.

http://www.omahasystem.org/shminter.htm

Individualize each one in the nursing orders.

Health Promotion in Group Nutrition

Intervention	Nursing Orders

Health Promotion in Group Physical Activity

Intervention	Nursing Orders

7. Describe how the roles of the community nurse are central to the implementation of these interventions.

_____

_____

_____

As part of the surveillance of individual outcomes, the nurse takes Javier on a home visit to an elderly Asian woman who is now 2 days home from short-term rehab after surgery to repair a broken hip. She lives at home with her spouse who is the primary caregiver during her recovery. She still requires the use of a walker and assistance with toileting, and help getting on and off the toilet. She is able to complete self-care that does not require standing/walking (bathing, eating). Screening during her acute care admission demonstrated severe osteoporosis. The interventions developed for the aggregate within the health department strategies were implemented during the rehabilitation phase and now continue. In addition she was prescribed alendronate sodium (Fosamax) 70 mg weekly 1 hour before breakfast. The patient was referred to the county home health services for assessment of the need for skilled nursing services.

8. How is the goal of home healthcare central to the needs of this referral?

9. Discuss the distinctive features of home healthcare that make visiting this patient different from a routine visit to a patient in an acute care facility.

_____

_____

_____

_____

10. Based on the Medicare definition of skilled nursing care, discuss whether this patient should qualify for services.

_____

_____

_____

_____

_____

_____

_____

_____

_____

_____

_____

11. Discuss the similarities and differences between a shift assessment in an acute care facility and an assessment in the home care environment.

_____

_____

_____

_____

_____

_____

_____

_____

12. One of the care components that the home care nurse identifies using the Clinical Care Classification (CCC) system is the Medication component related to the newly prescribed alendronate sodium (Fosamax) regimen. Write out a CCC nursing diagnosis and interventions to address this issue.

You may need to use your resources to learn about this medication and nursing implications related to educational needs and safe administration. In addition, information about the CCC and a complete list of diagnoses, outcomes, and interventions can be accessed by using the tables tab at this Web site:

http://www.sabacare.com/Tables/Components.html

_____

_____

_____

_____

_____

_____

_____

_____

_____

_____

_____

_____

_____

_____

_____

Ethics and Values

You are the charge nurse on a skilled nursing unit at the local long term-care facility caring for Mrs. Charlotte Boyer, an 91-year-old resident who had a stroke 6 months ago requiring placement in the facility. She requires assistance with hygiene and mobility needs, is unable to feed herself, has difficulty with speech and swallowing, and must be constantly monitored for aspiration. She has recently had an incident of aspiration pneumonia. Prior to this event she lived independently and was active in her community. For the past few days she has been refusing her meals, becoming agitated and angry during feedings. The primary care provider has recommended placement of a PEG tube for enteral feedings to maintain an adequate nutritional status. Her son is in favor of the feeding tube and states, "Not feeding mother is cruel and the tube is the right thing to do. Not feeding mother is almost like killing her. I do not think we should play God." The daughter is ambivalent about the feeding tube in that she is aware that her mother would not have wanted any artificial measures, including a feeding tube, to keep her alive. In addition, she feels that her mother's decision to refuse food indicates an attempt to be in control of her own life. She states, "I think I know how she feels and it's almost like the golden rule—do unto others as you would have them do unto you." The children share the power of attorney and power of healthcare for their mother. They have asked you to help them work through this decision-making process and the daughter states, "We need a tie-breaker, as we are at odds as to what to do."

1. Discuss why changes in societal factors have contributed to the frequency of ethical problems for nurses in today's healthcare environment.

_____

_____

_____

_____

_____

_____

_____

_____

_____

_____

_____

_____

_____

_____

_____

_____

_____

2. Discuss how each of the following concepts is integral to this patient care situation:
a. Autonomy:

_____

_____

_____

_____

_____

_____

_____

_____

_____

_____

_____

_____

_____

_____

b. Nonmaleficence:

_____

_____

_____

_____

_____

_____

_____

_____

c. Beneficence:

_____

_____

_____

_____

_____

_____

_____

_____

_____

d. Veracity:

_____

_____

_____

_____

_____

_____

3. Based on the comments/perspectives of each of the adult children, identify which Kohlberg's stage of moral development is being exhibited by each. Explain.

_____

_____

_____

_____

_____

_____

_____

_____

_____

_____

_____

_____

_____

_____

_____

_____

_____

_____

_____

_____

_____

4. Using the descriptions of the terms, describe your own beliefs, attitudes, and values regarding this situation.

_____

_____

_____

_____

_____

_____

_____

_____

_____

_____

_____

_____

_____

_____

_____

_____

_____

_____

_____

_____

_____

_____

_____

_____

_____

5. Discuss how the moral framework of Ethics of Care would direct your approach to this care issue.

_____

_____

_____

_____

_____

_____

_____

_____

_____

_____

_____

_____

6. How does the American Nurses Association Code of Ethics or the Canadian Association Code of Ethics provide a foundation for ethical decision-making in this situation?

_____

_____

_____

_____

_____

_____

_____

7. Using the assessment/analysis step of the nursing process, describe the problem and alternative approaches for this situation.

8. Next, use the MORAL Model to work through the situation to come up with alternative approaches for this family situation.

9. As an advocate, your first priority is the patient. You have identified the nursing diagnosis of Moral Distress[†] for this patient. What defining characteristics are present in this situation?

_____

_____

10. The NOC outcome of Personal Autonomy is identified. Discuss your role as patient advocate in this situation and determine appropriate NIC interventions that encompass the needs of both the patient and family.

_____

_____

_____

_____

_____

_____

_____

_____

_____

_____

_____

_____

_____

_____

_____

_____

_____

_____

_____

_____

_____

_____

Legal Issues

Clinical practice is a process closely regulated by legal parameters to ensure safety of both the patients and the practitioners. Knowledge of the laws and regulations is vital to every nurse in practice to protect all parties involved in our complex health-care delivery systems. The parameters that guide professional practice also guide your practice as a nursing student.

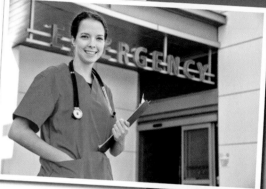

Betsy Sellars, a nursing student, has been assigned by the clinical instructor to assist in the care of the following patients during her clinical rotation in the Emergency Department at the local hospital:

- 42-year-old female who is unresponsive secondary to a narcotic overdose
- 2-month-old female with scald burns to lower extremities
- 91-year-old male with urosepsis/malnutrition
- 24-year-old female with suspected ectopic pregnancy

1. Discuss the importance of each of the following regulations in the provision of care to patients in this setting:
   a. Health Insurance Portability and Accountability Act (HIPAA)
   b. Emergency Medical Treatment and Active Labor Act (EMTALA)
   c. Patient Self Determination Act (PSDA)

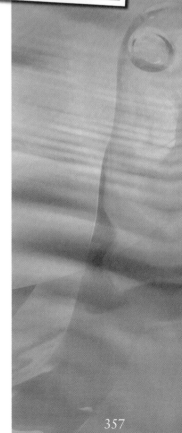

HIPAA	
EMTALA	
PSDA	

2. Which of the admitted patients should be considered within the mandatory reporting laws? Discuss your rationale for your choice(s).

_____

_____

_____

_____

_____

_____

_____

_____

_____

_____

_____

The 24-year-old is an acquaintance Betsy knows from church and she is surprised to see the admitting diagnosis. Beginning the admission assessment with the assigned RN, Betsy comments, "Hi Kelly, we are here to assess what is happening so that you can get the best care. It doesn't matter what the diagnosis is, and I was telling the nurse here that you are not that kind of girl."

3. Discuss whether the elements of defamation of character are present in this situation.

_____

_____

_____

_____

_____

The patient admitted with urosepsis and malnutrition is slightly confused. He knows who he is and why he is in the hospital, but not what day it is. He wants to go home and does not see that it is necessary for him to stay. He has been stabilized and is scheduled for admission to the medical unit. He frequently attempts to get up off the ED bed and the staff is concerned for his safety. The orderly, showing a waist restraint to the patient says, "Mr. Wells, if you continue we are going to have to put a restraint belt on you and tie you down so you can't get up."

4. Can this action by the orderly be interpreted as an intentional tort in a court of law? Why or why not?

Orders are received for the care of the 2-month-old with burn injuries. The skin is cleansed and dressed per protocol and the child is to be admitted to the pediatric unit. The parent has decided against admission for the child and communicates to leave AMA (against medical advice). The parent states that she is able to care for the child at home and requests instructions for care of the burns.

5. How should the nurse handle this situation including aspects of informed consent regarding leaving AMA? Consider the elements of informed consent normally used in the healthcare setting.

...

After the patient with the narcotic overdose receives naxolone (Narcan), she is more awake but is now vomiting. An order is received for gastrointestinal intubation. The ED nurse asks Betsy to place the NG tube, to which she replies, "I've never done that before—I've just read about it." The ED preceptor assures her that she will help her through the procedure. The ED nurse tells the patient that the physician ordered the tube "to help with the vomiting." The patient requested medication instead of an NG tube to help with the vomiting. Without consulting with the ED physician, the nurse tells the patient that the doctor does not want to order any more drugs that might interact with the medications she had already taken. The patient reluctantly agrees to the tube placement. Betsy's first attempt is unsuccessful because of the patient's forceful gagging. On the second try the tube goes into place. The ED nurse verifies placement by auscultating an air bolus over the epigastric region. The patient complains, "It feels awful—I feel like I can't breathe—please take it out." The ED nurse assures the patient that it is a common feeling to have after an NG tube is placed. Twenty minutes later the patient is exhibiting respiratory distress and the abdominal x-ray for tube placement shows the nasogastric tube lodged in the right bronchus. This subsequently resulted in a pneumothorax (collapsed lung due to a puncture) requiring a chest tube. The NG tube is immediately removed but the patient continues to have respiratory compromise resulting in the need for endotracheal intubation and mechanical ventilation. The ED physician states, "She was going to need that anyway because of the amount of narcotics in her system—I didn't think the Narcan would take care of it all." Afterward, the patient is transferred to the ICU for further care. She recovers from this event and is transferred to a private psychiatric clinic for follow-up.

Six months later, the hospital, the ED staff, as well as the nursing student are named in a malpractice suit by this patient. She is suing for damages related to false imprisonment, enforced hospitalization, and the nasogastric intubation procedure with subsequent need for a chest tube that resulted in an insertion scar. The patient is a swimsuit model and this has negatively affected her employment opportunities.

6. Define the four elements necessary to prove a malpractice case and the aspects of this situation that indicate a "preponderance of evidence."

_____

_____

_____

_____

_____

Duty	Evidence
Duty: The legal responsibility of the nurse for assigned patients and their care	
Breach of duty: Occurs when the nurse fails to meet standards in providing care in a reasonable and prudent manner	
Causation: The breach of duty is the direct and proximate cause of the injury suffered by the patient	
Damages: Monetary award to remedy the harm suffered by the patient	

7. Using the steps of the nursing process, decide if there is a "preponderance of evidence" in the breach of duty to this patient. You may need to read/review the procedure and evidence-based practices for proper nasogastric intubation.

Step of the Nursing Process	Breach of Duty
Assessment/Analysis	
Diagnosis	

(Continued)

Step of the Nursing Process	Breach of Duty
Planning	
Implementation	
Evaluation	

8. How did Betsy violate professional standards in her student role in this situation?

_____

_____

_____

_____

_____

_____

_____

_____

_____

_____

_____

_____

_____

_____

_____

Index

A

Abdellah, Faye, 89
Acid-base disorder, 304
Activity and exercise, 261–267
  ambulation, 263–264
    body mechanics for safe patient care and
      transfers, 264
    communicating with physiatrist, 266–267
    diagnosis, outcomes, and goals, 265
    hazards of immobility, 261–262
    nursing interventions, 265
    positioning devices, 263
    range of motion exercises, 266
    regaining muscle strength, 263
    SBAR format, 266–267
    teaching to use crutches, 267
Admission assessment data, analyzing, 46, 54–55
  clusters, 47–49
  cues, 46–47
  diagnostic labels and etiological factors, 49–50
  gaps, 48
Advance directives, 143
Aging adults. See Elderly
AMA (leaving against medical advice), 359
Ambulation, 263–264
Ambulatory care, 14–15
American Nurses Association (ANA), 6–7, 13, 130
  Code of Ethics, 353
  Standards of Practice, 32–33, 57
Anxiety, 113–114
Apical and peripheral pulses, 162–163
Asepsis and preventing infection, 177–186, 289–290
  chain of infection, 178
  community setting, 186
  Critical-Thinking Model (CTM), 185
  diagnostic testing, 182
  infection control, 158
  infection control nurse, 185
  lifestyle factors, 179–181
  patient factors that increase risk of infection,
    181–182
  secondary defense indicators, 179
  standard precautions, 183
  tertiary defenses, 179
  types of specific immunity
    cell-mediated immunity, 179
    humoral immunity, 179
Authoritarian leadership style, 308
Autonomy, 350

B

Baseline, determining for inflating cuff to
  measure blood pressure, 161
Bathing/Hygiene Self-Care Deficit, 195
Baths, 195–196
Bed exit alarm, 189–190

Bedpans, 237
Behavioral theories of leadership, 308–309
Beneficence, 351
Benner's model of clinical skills and judgment, 12
BMI, 232
Body Image Enhancement intervention, 114
Body mechanics for safe patient care and transfers,
  264
BOHSE (Brief Oral Health Status Examination),
  197
Bowel elimination: constipation, 243–246
  digital removal of stool, 246
  factors affecting elimination, 244–245
  focused physical assessment, 244
    rectal exam, 244
  oil-retention enema, 245
  questioning patient, 243
  teaching healthy bowel routine, 246
Bowel elimination: diarrhea, 247–249
  diet, 248
  fecal occult blood test (FOBT), 248
  medication request, 248
  stool specimen, 247
Breach of duty, 361–362
Breast cancer, 141
Brief Oral Health Status Examination (BOHSE),
  197
Burn unit, 111–112

C

Calorie reduction, 232
CAM (complementary and alternative modalities),
  323–325
Canadian Nurses Association (CNA), 6–7, 13
  Code of Ethics, 353
Cardiac dysrhythmias, 294
Cardiac pump effectiveness, 294
Care and comfort, 87–88
Caregiver Role Strain, 123
Care plan modifications, 76–78
Caring, 19, 28
Causation (in malpractice), 361
CBE note, 153–154
CCC (Clinical Care Classification) system, 346–347
Cell-mediated immunity, 179
Chain of infection, 178
Change
  evaluating, 313
  implementing, 313
  resistance to, 310–312
Chest physiotherapy, 292
Children. See Growth and development
Chronic Pain diagnosis and outcomes, 257–258
Citations, research, 92–93
Clinical Care Classification (CCC) system, 346–347
Clusters, data, 47–49

Combivent inhaler extender or spacer, 207
Communication and therapeutic relationships, 165–170
    communication barriers, 168–169
    developmental stage, 165–166
    environment, 165–166
    gender, 165–166
    nonverbal communication, 166
    personal space, 165–166
    roles and relationships, 165–166
    SBAR format, 169–170
    sociocultural factors, 165–166
    techniques, 168
    therapist, communicating with, 169–170
    verbal communication, 166
Communication barriers, 168–169
Communication pattern and coping processes, 122
Community-acquired bacterial pneumonia, 291–292
Community-based care, 14–15, 186, 341–347
    Clinical Care Classification (CCC) system, 346–347
    Healthy People 2020, 341–342
    home healthcare, 345–346
        diagnoses, outcomes, and interventions, 346–347
    Omaha Problem Classification Scheme, 343–344
    osteoporosis, 341–347
Complementary and alternative modalities (CAM), 323–325
Conflict resolution, 314–315
Confusion, perfusion and, 295
Continuing education, 11
Continuous cardiac monitoring, nursing responsibilities, 293
Coping. *See* Stress-coping-adaptation
CPAP treatment, 275
Crisis intervention, 223
Critical thinking and the nursing process, 19–29
    caring, 19, 28
    characteristics of a critical thinker, 20
        life skill as well as nursing skill, 20
    critical thinking, definition of (Heaslip), 19
    critical-thinking problem, 20–23
    full-spectrum nursing, 29
    model for critical thinking, 24–27
        analyzing assumptions, 26
        considering alternatives, 25–26
        contextual awareness, 25
        inquiry, 25
        reflecting/making a decision, 26–27
    nurse-patient dyad, 29
    nursing knowledge, 27
    nursing process, 28
        critical thinking and, 28
    today's healthcare delivery system, 23
Critical-Thinking Model (CTM), 185
Crutches, teaching to use, 267
Cues, recognizing, 46–47
    changes in usual behaviors, 47
    changes in usual health patterns, 47
    delayed growth and development, 47
    deviation from population norms, 46
    nonproductive of dysfunctional behavior, 47
Culture and ethnicity, 127–133
    cultural assessment, 133
    Cultural Brokerage, 131
    cultural sensitivity and competence, 129–130
    designating on health record, 128
    Hmong culture, 127–128
    influences on plan of care, 128–129
        communication, 129
        social organization, 129
        space, 129
        time orientation, 129
    language barriers, 132
    nursing diagnoses, 130
    socialization, acculturation, and assimilation, 127

D

Damages (in malpractice), 361
Data clusters, 47–49
Data gaps, 48
Deductive reasoning, 89
Defamation of character, 358
Defense mechanisms, 221
Deficient fluid volume, 297–298
    prevention, 300
Deficient knowledge nursing diagnosis, 214
Delegating activities to nursing assistive personnel (NAP), 85
    "Five Rights of Delegation," 85
Delegating interventions to UAPs
    skin integrity, 286
Democratic leadership style, 309
Dentures, 198
Depression, 114–116
Developmental stage, 112. *See also* Growth and development
    communication and, 165–166
    teaching and, 213
Diabetes, 193
Diet
    diarrhea, 248
    instruction, 232
    vegetarian, 233
Digital removal of stool, 246
Disturbed Sleep Pattern diagnosis, 276
Diversity, 5
DNAR order, 143
Documenting and reporting, 86, 149–155
    assessment, 39–40
    CBE note, 153–154
    communicating inadequate pain medication/ schedule to primary care provider, 155
    electronic health record (EHR), 152–153
    focus note (DAR), 153, 155
    graphic record, 149
    intake and output, 150
    interpreting reports, 150–151
    mandatory reporting laws, 358

medication administration record, 150
nursing admission data form, 149
organizing patient data into PACE format, 152
questioning primary care provider orders, 155
SBAR format, 155
source-oriented and problem-oriented records, 153
using documentation, 73
using professional terms, 151
Dosage calculation, 207
Down syndrome, 171–175
Dressings, 282–285
Duty (in malpractice), 361
Dying. *See* Loss, grief, and dying

E

Education
continuing, 11
pathways for registered nurse (RN), 10–11
socialization, 11
EE (eosinophilic esophagitis), 211
EHRs (electronic health records), 152–153, 319
Elderly, 101–103
exercise, 101
incorporating Erickson's developmental theory and the task stage, 103
physical assessment, 102
sexuality and, 272
socialization, 101
Electrolyte imbalance, 302–303
breathing, 303
hypocalcemia, 303–304
Electronic health records (EHRs), 152–153, 319
Electronic mail, 318
Electronic mail (Listserv), 318
Elimination, bowel. *See* Bowel elimination, constipation; Bowel elimination, diarrhea
Elimination: urinary, 235–240
"at risk" diagnoses, 236
bedpans, 237
facilitating voiding, 240
indwelling catheter, 237–239
care of, 239
preparing patient for procedure, 238
prevention/surveillance for urinary tract infections, 240
removing, 239
repositioning patient in bed, 239
selection of type, 237
Urinary incontinence, functional (diagnosis), 236
Emergency Medical Treatment and Active Labor Act (EMTALA), 357–358
Emotional intelligence, 309
Eosinophilic esophagitis (EE), 211
Erickson's Psychosocial Development Theory, 90, 101, 103
Ethics and values, 349–355
American Nurses Association Code of Ethics, 353
autonomy, 350

beneficence, 351
Canadian Association Code of Ethics, 353
Ethics of Care, 353
Kohlberg's stage of moral development, 351
Moral Distress, 355
MORAL Model, 354
nonmaleficence, 351
patient advocate role, 355
Personal Autonomy, 355
societal factors, 350
veracity, 351
Eustress, 220
Evidence-based practice, 91
Examination, techniques of, 34
Exercise. *See* Activity and exercise
Extended care facilities, 14–15
Eye drop technique, 206

F

Falls, 187–191
Family, 119–125
Caregiver Role Strain, 123
communication pattern and coping processes, 122
definition of, 119
Family Interactional Theory, 121
family nursing approaches, 120
family as context for care, 120
family as system, 120
family as unit of care, 120
Family Processes, Interrupted, 122–123
health beliefs, 121
NIC interventions, 123
NOC outcomes, 123
resources, 123
structure, 120
Family Interactional Theory, 121
Family Processes, Interrupted, 122–123
Family Resiliency outcome, 145
Fecal occult blood test (FOBT), 248
Five Rights of Delegation, 85
right circumstance, 85
right communication, 85
right person, 85
right supervision, 85
right task, 85
Flow-oriented incentive spirometry, 338
Fluid, electrolyte, and acid-base balance, 297–304
acid-base disorder, 304
deficient fluid volume, 297–298
prevention, 300
electrolyte imbalance, 302–303
breathing, 303
hypocalcemia, 303–304
Fluid Volume Excess diagnosis, 300–301
gravity infusion, 298
increasing fluid intake, 300
intravenous site
catheter size, 299

finding vein, 299
  tattoo and, 299
  questioning primary physician orders, 301
FOBT (fecal occult blood test), 248
Focus note (DAR), 153, 155
Followership, 306
Full code, CPR delegation and, 295
Full-spectrum nursing model, 3–4, 29, 32, 67

G
Gaps in data, 48
Gender, 5, 112
  communication and, 165–166
"Get Up and Go Test," 191
Goal statements, 61
  collaborative problems, 61
Gordon's Functional Health Patterns, 38–39
Graphic record, 149
Gravity infusion, 298
Grieving, 142, 145. *See also* Loss, grief, and dying
Growth and development, 95–103
  elderly, 101–103
    exercise, 101
    incorporating Erickson's developmental
      theory and the task stage, 103
    physical assessment, 102
    socialization, 101
  health issues, 96
  middle school, 97–101
    appropriate issue for initial session with this
      group, 100
    incorporating major psychological tasks
      (Erickson) of adolescence into teaching/
      learning strategies, 101
  6 to 12 months, 96
  variations in, 95–96

H
Health and illness, 105–109
  having someone "in your corner," 109
  hip replacement, 105
  part of admission process rather than object of
    admission, 108
  rehabilitation, 105
  stage of illness behavior, 106
Health assessment, 173
  developmental stage, 171–175
    deferring aspects of full physical assessment,
      173–174
    explaining techniques of physical examination,
      172–173
  documenting data, 175
  equipment needed, 174–175
Health education, 330
Health history, 35–37
Health Insurance Portability and Accountability
  Act (HIPAA), 357–358
Health literacy, 213
Health promotion, 327–330
  assessment, 329

health education, 330
health protection and, 327
Pender's Health Promotion Model, 328
programs, 328
role modeling, 330
support for lifestyle change, 330
wellness diagnoses, outcomes, and interventions,
  330
Healthy People 2020, 341–342
Heaslip's definition of critical thinking, 19
Henderson, Virginia, 89
HIPAA (Health Insurance Portability and
  Accountability Act), 357–358
Hip replacement, 105
Hmong culture, 127–128
Holism, 323–325
  complementary and alternative modalities
    (CAM), 323–325
  Readiness for enhanced sleep (diagnosis),
    324
Home healthcare, 14–15, 345–346
  diagnoses, outcomes, and interventions,
    346–347
Homes-Rahe Social Readjustment Scale, 220
HOPE assessment tool, 136–137
Hospice care, 119, 141–146
Humoral immunity, 179
Hydraulic lift, moving patients without,
  198–199
Hygiene. *See* Self-care ability: hygiene
Hypocalcemia, 303–304

I
ICN (International Council of Nurses), 6–7,
  13
Immobility, hazards, 261–262
Impaired gas exchange diagnosis and outcomes,
  292
Impaired Tissue Integrity versus Impaired Skin
  Integrity diagnoses, 285
Inappropriate sexual behavior, 272
Inductive reasoning, 89
Indwelling catheter, 237–239
  care of, 239
  preparing patient for procedure, 238
  prevention/surveillance for urinary tract
    infections, 240
  removing, 239
  repositioning patient in bed, 239
  selection of type, 237
Infection. *See* Asepsis and preventing infection
Informatics, 317–322
  credibility of Web sites, 320–322
  EHRs, 319
  electronic mail (Listserv), 318
  integration with the nursing process, 317
  social networking, 318
  telehealth, 318
  text messaging, 318
  Web conferencing, 318
  webinars, 318

Injections
    minimizing discomfort, 208
    sites, 207
International Council of Nurses (ICN), 6–7, 13
Intravenous sites
    catheter size, 299
    finding vein, 299
    tattoo and, 299

K
Kohlberg's stages of moral development, 351

L
Laissez-faire leadership style, 309
Language barriers, 132
Laws, 12–13
Leading and management, 305–315
    behavioral theories, 308–309
    conflict resolution, 314–315
    evaluating change, 313
    followership and, 306
    implementing change, 313
    leadership styles, 308–309
        transactional, 309
        transformational, 309
    power, 307
    resistance to change, 310–312
    skills, 306
Learning. See Teaching and learning
Leaving against medical advice (AMA), 359
Legal issues, 357–362
    defamation of character, 358
    Emergency Medical Treatment and Active
        Labor Act (EMTALA), 357–358
    Health Insurance Portability and Accountability
        Act (HIPAA), 357–358
    leaving against medical advice (AMA), 359
    malpractice, 360–362
        breach of duty, 361–362
        causation, 361
        damages, 361
        duty, 361
    mandatory reporting laws, 358
    Patient Self Determination Act (PSDA),
        357–358
    professional standards, 362
    restraints, 359
Leninger, 130
Listserv, 318
Literature, reading analytically, 93–94
Literature, searching, 92–93
Long- versus short-term care, 58–59
Loss, grief, and dying, 141–146
    advance directives, 143
    care for the nurse, 146
    DNAR order, 143
    Family Resiliency outcome, 145
    Grieving, 142, 145
    hospice care, 141–146
    nursing diagnoses, 142–143
    postmortem care, 144

    supporting family, 144
    terminal illness, 141

M
Malnutrition, 228–229
Malpractice, 360–362
    breach of duty, 361–362
    causation, 361
    damages, 361
    duty, 361
Management. See Leading and Management
Mandatory reporting laws, 358
Maslow's Hierarchy of Needs, 38–39, 71–72, 90,
    113–114
    prioritizing problems by, 50–51
Measurement scales, 62–63
Medical diagnosis, problems with using, 44
Medication administration, 201–209
    applying patch when previous patch is still
        there, 206
    Combivent inhaler extender or spacer, 207
    communicating problems to primary care
        provider, 203
    dosage calculation, 207
    equipment needed, 203–204
    eye drop technique, 206
    information needed from previous shift nurse,
        201
    injection site, 207
    Medication Administration Record (MAR),
        150, 202
    minimizing injection discomfort, 208
    physical assessments and lab data, 203–204
    Rights of Medication, 204
    SBAR format, 203
    stock supply and unit dose systems, 202
    swallowing issues, 205
    syringe type and needle gauge, 207
    "Three Checks," 204
    unavailable medication, 205
Middle school age, 97–101
    appropriate issue for initial session with this
        group, 100
    incorporating major psychological tasks
        (Erickson) of adolescence into teaching/
        learning strategies, 101
Montgomery straps, 283
Moral Distress, 355
MORAL Model, 354
Morbidly obese patient, 193–199
Morse Fall Scale, 187
Muscle strength, regaining, 263
MyPlate strategy, 232–233

N
NANDA taxonomy (labels), 51–53, 65
Nasogastric feeding tubes, 229–231
    aspiration precautions, 231–232
    checking for placement, 231
"Never events," 188
NG irrigation, 337

NIC (Nursing Intervention Classification), 65
Nightingale, Florence, 3
Nightmares, 276
Nonmaleficence, 351
Nonverbal communication, 166
Nurse-patient dyad, 29
Nurses Improving Care for Healthsystem Elders
  (NICHE), 253
Nursing admission data form, 149
Nursing Intervention Classification (NIC), 65
Nursing orders
  prioritizing, 71–72
  writing, 70–71
Nursing process: assessment, 31–41
  ANA *Standards of Practice,* 32–33
  documentation, 39–40
  examination, techniques of, 34
  follow-up, 41
  four features of assessment, 31
  health history, 35–37
  importance to other steps of nursing process, 32
  information sources, 33
  organizing data, 38–40
    Gordon's Functional Health Patterns, 38–39
    Maslow's Hierarchy of Needs, 38–39
  overview, 31
  special needs assessment, 33
  validating conclusions, 37–38
Nursing process: evaluation, 73–78
  care plan modifications needed, 76–78
  documentation, using, 73
  essential to all aspects of patient care, 73
  goal achievement status, 75
  in long-term care facility, 74
  reassessment data, using, 74–75
Nursing process: implementation, 79–86
  delegating activities to nursing assistive
    personnel (NAP), 85
    "Five Rights of Delegation," 85
  documentation, 86
  explaining activities to patient, 82–84
  feedback points, 84
  grouping activities, 82
  knowledge/skills needed, 79–81
Nursing process: nursing diagnosis, 43–55
  analyzing admission assessment data, 46,
    54–55
    clusters, 47–49
    cues, 46–47
    diagnostic labels and etiological factors,
      49–50
    gaps, 48
  collaborative problem, 52
  determining, 44
  etiologies, 52
  five types, 44–46
    actual, 45
    possible, 45
    potential, 45
    syndrome, 46
    wellness (health promotion), 46

helps to validate nursing as a profession, 43
  importance to development of plan of care, 43
  NANDA-I Taxonomy II: Domains, Classes
    and Diagnoses (Labels), 51–53
  patient preference and, 51
  prioritizing problems by Maslow's Hierarchy
    of Needs and problem urgency, 50–51
  problems with using the medical diagnosis, 44
  quality, judging, 52–53
  self-knowledge and, 51
  verifying problems identified and contributing
    factors, 50
  writing diagnoses, 51–53
Nursing process: planning interventions, 65–72
  activities, identifying, 68–69
  factors to consider in meeting goals, 66
  full-spectrum nursing model, 67
  interventions, identifying, 67–68
  nursing orders
    prioritizing, 71–72
    writing, 70–71
  overview, 65
  parts of diagnostic statement and possible
    interventions, 66
  resources, 66
Nursing process: planning outcomes, 57–63
  evaluation, 63
  four kinds of care, 58
  goal statements, 61
    collaborative problems, 61
  identifying outcome and indicators for
    diagnoses, 62
  learning needs, 63
  measurement scales, 62–63
  ongoing process, 57
  roadmap of patient care, 57
  short- versus long-term care, 58–59
  standardized care plans, 59–60
    individualizing, 60
Nursing profession and practice, 1–15
  American Nurses Association (ANA), 6–7, 13
  Canadian Nurses Association (CNA), 6–7, 13
  clinical skills and judgment (Benner's model), 12
  definition of nursing profession, 5–7
  diversity, 5
  education
    continuing education, 11
    pathways for registered nurse (RN), 10–11
    socialization, 11
  exit competency for your program of study, 12
  "full-spectrum nursing," 3–4
  gender, 5
  International Council of Nurses (ICN), 6–7, 13
  laws, 12–13
  Nightingale, Florence, 3
  perceptions of, 2–3, 10
  practice settings, 14–15
    ambulatory care, 14–15
    community health, 14–15
    extended care facilities, 14–15
    home care, 14–15

as a profession, discipline, and occupation, 9–10
  purposes of nursing care, 14
  race and ethnicity, 5
  roles and functions of nurses, 8–9
  societal and healthcare trends, 15
  standards of practice, 12–13
Nursing theory, 87–90
  care and comfort, 87–88
  deductive reasoning, 89
  Faye Abdellah, 89
  inductive reasoning, 89
  reasoning, importance of, 88–89
  theories from other disciplines, 90
    Erickson's Psychosocial Development Theory, 90
    Maslow's Hierarchy of Human Needs, 90
    Selye's Stress and Adaptation Theory, 90
  Virginia Henderson, 89
Nutrition, 227–234
  BMI, 232
  calorie reduction, 232
  dementia, 230
  dietary instruction, 232
  dyspnea, 228
  independence during meals, 232
  malnutrition, 228–229
  MyPlate strategy, 232–233
  nasogastric feeding tubes, 229–231
    aspiration precautions, 231–232
    checking for placement, 231
  sodium restriction, 232, 234
  stimulating patient's appetite, 227
  vegetarian diet, 233
Nutritional status
  skin integrity and, 284

O

Obesity, 193–199
Oil-retention enema, 245
Omaha Problem Classification Scheme, 343–344
Osteoporosis, 341–347
Otic irrigation, 251–252
Oxygenation, 287–292
  chest physiotherapy, 292
  communicating with primary care provider, 292
  community-acquired bacterial pneumonia, 291–292
  Impaired gas exchange diagnosis and outcomes, 292
  older adults, 287
  preventing spread of infection, 289–290
  pulse oximetry reading, obtaining, 288
  purified protein derivative (PPD) tests, 290
  SBAR format, 292
  smoking cessation, 288–289
  sputum specimens, obtaining, 288
  teaching to enhance mobilization of secretions, 289

P

PACE format, 152
PACU, 334–339
Pain management, 253–259
  Chronic Pain diagnosis and outcomes, 257–258
  communicating problems to surgeon, 254
  factors influencing pain experience, 253
  interventions, 256
  nonpharmacological pain relief measures, 259
  PCA, 255
    amitriptyline, 256
    naloxene and, 255
    patient teaching, 255
    placebos, 257
  responding to patient medication request, 253
  SBAR format, 354
Pain medication
  falls and, 188–189
Parish nurses, 95
Patch, applying when previous patch is still there, 206
Patient advocate role, 355
Patient Safety Goals, 334
Patient Self Determination Act (PSDA), 357–358
PCA, 255
  amitriptyline, 256
  naloxene and, 255
  patient teaching, 255
  placebos, 257
Pender's Health Promotion Model, 328
Penrose drain, 283
Percutaneous endoscopic gastrostomy (PEG), 211
Perfusion, 293–295
  cardiac dysrhythmias, 294
  cardiac pump effectiveness, 294
  confusion and, 295
  continuous cardiac monitoring, nursing responsibilities, 293
  full code, CPR delegation and, 295
  reassuring patient, 294
Perineal care, 197
Perioperative nursing, 331–339
  admission nursing assessment history, 331–332
  PACU, 334–339
  Patient Safety Goals, 334
  post-operative phase, 334–339
    flow-oriented incentive spirometry, 338
    NG irrigation, 337
    preventing complications, 338–339
  pre-operative teaching, 333
  psychosocial needs, 333
  questioning preoperative orders, 332
  World Health Organization (WHO) Surgical Safety Checklist, 334
Peripheral pulses, 162–163
Personal Autonomy, 355
Personal space, 165–166
Physiatrist, communicating with, 266–267
PICO acronym, 92
PLISSIT model, 270

Positioning devices, 263
Postmortem care, 144
Post-operative phase, 334–339
  flow-oriented incentive spirometry, 338
  hip surgery patients, 177–186
  NG irrigation, 337
  preventing complications, 338–339
Power, 307
PPD (purified protein derivative) tests, 290
Practice settings, 14–15
  ambulatory care, 14–15
  community health, 14–15
  extended care facilities, 14–15
  home care, 14–15
Praying for clients, 140
Pre-operative teaching, 333
Problem-oriented records, 153
Professional standards, 362
Professional terms, using, 151
PSDA (Patient Self Determination Act), 357–358
Psychosocial health and illness, 111–117
  anxiety, 113–114
  Body Image Enhancement intervention, 114
  depression, 114–116
  developmental level, 112
  gender, 112
  health histories, 116–117
  internal influences, 112
  psychosocial influences, 111–112
  relationships, 112
  self-concept, 112–113
  suicide risk and prevention, 115
Pulse oximetry reading, obtaining, 288
Purified protein derivative (PPD) tests, 290
Purnell, 130
Pyrexia, 162

Q
Quantitative versus qualitative research, 92

R
Race and ethnicity, 5
Range of motion exercises, 266
Readiness for Enhanced Coping (diagnosis), 224
Readiness for enhanced sleep (diagnosis), 324
Reasoning, importance of, 88–89
Reassessment data, using, 74–75
Rectal exam, 244
Rehabilitation, 105
Religion. See Spirituality
Reminiscence therapy for persons with dementia, 91–92
Reporting. See Documenting and Reporting
Research, 91–94
  evidence-based practice, 91
  formulating searchable questions using PICO acronym, 92
  quantitative versus qualitative research, 92
  reading the literature analytically, 93–94
  reminiscence therapy for persons with dementia, 91–92
  searching the literature, 92–93

Resistance to change, 310–312
Respirations, 162
Rest. See Sleep and rest
Restraints, 359
Rights of Medication, 204
Risk for falls diagnosis, 188
Roadmap of patient care, 57

S
SBAR format, 155, 169–170, 203, 266–267, 271, 277, 292, 354
Secondary defense indicators, 179
Self-care ability: hygiene, 193–199
  Bathing/Hygiene Self-Care Deficit, 195
  baths, 195–196
  Brief Oral Health Status Examination (BOHSE), 197
  decreasing skin problems, 197
  dentures, 198
  effects of health status, 193, 195
  interviewing patient, 194
  moving patient without hydraulic lift, 198–199
  perineal care, 197
  willingness and ability to perform ADLs, 194
Selye's Stress and Adaptation Theory, 90
Sensory perception, 249–252
  assessments, 251
  communication with hearing impairment, 252
  developmental variation, 250
  medical problems' effect upon, 249
  otic irrigation, 251–252
  outcome and goals, 251
  personality and lifestyle, 250
  sensory overload/deprivation, 250
Sexual health, 269–272
  aging adults, sexuality and, 272
  communicating with primary care provider, 271
  health and illness factors, 270
  inappropriate sexual behavior, 272
  open-ended questions, 270
  patient teaching for sildenafil, 272
  PLISSIT model, 270
  SBAR format, 271
  sexual counseling, 270
  Sexual Dysfunction diagnosis and outcomes, 270
  sexual history, 269
Short- versus long-term care, 58–59
Sildenafil, patient teaching for, 272
Skin integrity, 197, 279–286
  delegating interventions to UAP, 286
  dressings, 282–285
  equipment, 283
    Montgomery straps, 283
    Penrose drain, 283
  factors affecting, 280–281
  Impaired Tissue Integrity versus Impaired Skin Integrity diagnoses, 285
  nutritional status and, 284
  wound characteristics, 281–282
  Wound Healing, Secondary Intention (outcome), 286
  wound irrigation, 283

Sleep and rest, 275–277
  communicating with primary care provider for
    medication, 277
  difficulty getting in hospital setting, 275
  Disturbed Sleep Pattern diagnosis, 276
  measuring quality after implementation of nurs-
    ing interventions, 277
  nightmares, 276
  nursing interventions, 276–277
  SBAR format, 277
Smoking cessation, 288–289
Social networking, 318
Societal factors, 350
Sodium restriction, 232, 234
Source-oriented and problem-oriented records,
  153
Space, 129
Special needs assessment, 33
Spirituality, 135–140
  barriers to spiritual care, 135
  HOPE assessment tool
    assessment, 136–137
  praying for clients, 140
  spiritual assessment, 136–137
  Spiritual Distress diagnosis, 137–138
    interventions, 139–140
Sputum specimens, obtaining, 288
Stage of illness behavior, 106
Standardized care plans, 59–60
  individualizing, 60
Standard precautions, 183
Standards of practice, 12–13
Stock supply and unit dose systems, 202
Stool, digital removal of, 246
Stress-coping-adaptation, 219–225
  Coping Enhancement intervention, 224
  crisis intervention, 223
  defense mechanisms, 221
  health promotion, 225
  Homes-Rahe Social Readjustment Scale, 220
  outcomes, 224
  personal factors, 222
  Readiness for Enhanced Coping diagnosis, 224
  stressors, identifying, 220–221
Suicide, 115
Swallowing issues, 205
Syringe type and needle gauge, 207

T
Tattoo and intravenous sites, 299
Teaching and learning, 211–217
  assessment data, 213–214
  Deficient knowledge nursing diagnosis, 214
  developmental stage, 213

  evaluating goals, 217
  goals and learning domains, 214
  health literacy, 213
  learning ability, 212
  teaching plan, 215–216
Teaching plan, 215–216
Telehealth, 318
Temperature assessment, site for, 160
Terminal illness, 141
Tertiary defenses, 179
Text messaging, 318
Therapeutic relationships, communication
  and. See Communication and therapeutic
  relationships
"Three Checks," 204
Time orientation, 129
Transactional leadership style, 309
Transformational leadership style, 309

U
UAP, working with, 164, 286
Urinary incontinence, functional (diagnosis), 236

V
Values. See Ethics and values
Vegetarian diet, 233
Veracity, 351
Verbal communication, 166
Vital signs, 157–164
  apical and peripheral pulses, 162–163
  baseline, determining for inflating cuff to
    measure blood pressure, 161
  expected values, 157–158
  facility equipment, 158
  factors affecting, 158–161
  infection control, 158
  nursing diagnoses, outcomes, and interventions,
    161–162
  pyrexia, 162
  respirations, 162
  site (oral, rectal, axillary) for assessing
    temperature, 160
  UAP, working with, 164
Voiding, facilitating, 240

W
Web conferencing, 318
Webinars, 318
Web sites
  credibility of, 320–322
World Health Organization (WHO) Surgical
  Safety Checklist, 334
Wound care, 279–286. See also Skin integrity